CONTENT

DISCLAIMER

This book is based on the lectures and studies of Barbara O'Neill, providing insights into health and wellness. While it offers advice, it is not a substitute for professional medical guidance. Readers should consult with healthcare professionals for personalized advice on their health. The author and publisher are not responsible for any consequences resulting from the use of the information in this book.

Published by Lane Snyder

INTRODUCTION

Can you picture a life where you're free from the daily burdens, both physical and mental, and instead, thriving with amazing health, vitality, and incredible energy? Do you ever feel overwhelmed by the sheer volume of advice, without a clear roadmap, leaving you uncertain about the right foods to eat or lifestyle choices to make for a healthier path?

If you answered yes to both questions, then I suggest you keep reading, as your worries and uncertainties will come to an end. In today's life, we are bombarded with unnatural foods and objects, and most of us lead very unnatural lives, contrary to the principles of health. Even those who aspire to live better and maintain a great, healthy lifestyle often encounter sickness, stress, anxiety, and skin problems. Thanks to Barbara O'Neill's studies, we now have a guide and a roadmap of unique remedies for a healthy lifestyle.

Her teachings not only provide us with a better understanding of the human body and help us make better choices in our everyday lives but also offer precise recommendations on what to do, what to eat, and what to drink for healing. This book will guide you through her teachings, delivering not only theoretical advice but, more importantly, practical insights for a better life.

She explains that our bodies are incredible self-healing machines, constantly renewing themselves based on the instructions in our DNA. Therefore, if we give to our body the right inputs and we live in a healthy and natural environment we heal, because we are meant to conduct healthy lives. Think about it—our eyes make new cells every one to two days, our skin refreshes every month, bones renew every three months, and the liver regenerates every six weeks. In about two years, we essentially get a brand-new body.

This means that daily choices and our routines affect our body and life drastically. We can become completely new people. If we struggle with anything, through daily choices we can massively change and improve our conditions. Following this book you will learn how to change your life and you will exceed your expectations.

This book will guide you through several teachings and you will find out many things that are extremely good and bad for you. body. Thanks to Barbara's teachings you will achieve a new level of health.
In the pages of this book, you will find a comprehensive compilation of the teachings of Barbara O'Neill. After attending her captivating lectures and exploring the profound insights in her books, the main topics have been carefully selected and developed. Her eloquence and wisdom have left a lasting impression on readers, offering an illuminating perspective on crucial themes that permeate everyday life. This collection aims to make accessible and share with the reader the key concepts that emerged during Barbara O'Neill's lectures, thus creating an engaging and informative journey through which to delve into her valuable teachings.

Many chapters and topics will be addressed over the next pages. I'll give you a little example of something that can be implemented today. There are several routines that Barbara started that changed her life drastically. Going to sleep early, waking up at 5 AM has become the norm, allowing her to experience the tranquillity of dawn. A brisk walk at 6 AM is her daily commitment to health, energizing both body and mind. By 7 AM, a hearty breakfast becomes more than a meal. Exercising every day and Consuming an alkaline based diet are also key for her health.

Living naturally and in an environment that maximize our potential is the key for a long and healthy life. People who live in Blue Zones, represent communities with high life expectancy. Therefore, Barbara studied people who live the longest and she found out that the people who live the longest are :

- Okinawans, which is a Japanese island.

- Sardinians, people living on an Italian island.

- Seventh Day Adventists.

The common denominators among these groups of people include the following:

1. They maintain an active lifestyle : Engaging in daily exercises regardless of their fitness levels. Notably, their physical activity is not confined to structured workouts but extends to activities like walks and embracing a natural and primitive lifestyle, aligning with the way humans are naturally meant to live.

2. Eat natural food : Their dietary habits revolve around consuming food in its natural state, primarily following a vegetarian diet. When meat is consumed, it is not a significant part of their daily intake. This might seem like common sense, but it holds crucial importance in today's world where many foods deviate from their natural origins.

3. They are highly social individuals : While this may seem apparent, contemporary life often involves fewer social interactions.

These common denominators will be thoroughly explained in the book.

This book brings together the valuable lessons she shares in her teachings and talks. It's like a go-to guide for a better life, offering straightforward advice on different aspects. Whether it's about life, health, or overall well-being, this book aims to make her insightful ideas easy to understand for everyone. It's designed to be a simple roadmap for a more fulfilling and enriched life.

FOUNDATIONS OF HEALTH

1. Pure Air:
Barbara O'Neill emphasizes the importance of breathing in clean, fresh air for overall well-being. She advocates spending time outdoors in areas with good air quality to support respiratory health and vitality.

2. Sunshine:
O'Neill recognizes the role of natural sunlight in the production of Vitamin D, essential for various bodily functions. She encourages safe sun exposure to maintain optimal health as the benefits are numerous.

3. Temperance:
Barbara O'Neill often discusses the impact of diet and lifestyle choices on health. She talks in favour of a balanced, alkaline diet, avoiding excessive consumption of acidic stimulants like caffeine and processed foods for a more harmonious internal environment. As well as making mindful choices.

4. Sleep:
O'Neill underscores the significance of sleep in her teachings. She promotes establishing healthy sleep patterns to support physical and mental restoration.

5. Exercising:
In O'Neill's holistic approach to health, exercise is definitely a key part. Exercising consistently enhances cardiovascular health, maintains flexibility, and supports overall well-being.

6. Avoid High-Carb diet:
She recommends a balanced diet with a mindful approach to carbohydrate intake, emphasising whole foods and nutritional balance.

7. Mental Health :

Mental health plays a key part in overall health. On top of much advice, she suggests mindfulness practices, stress reduction techniques, and positive thought patterns to support mental well-being in her holistic approach to health.

According to O'Neill's studies, the foundations of health serve as the crucial keys to a wholesome life, facilitating the optimization of well-being across physical, spiritual, emotional, and mental dimensions. These pillars are essential for everyone, regardless of age, ethnicity, gender, or fitness level. By dedicating efforts to enhance these life foundations, many issues can be effectively addressed, or even better, anticipated and prevented. It is crucial to understand these 'Foundations of Health,' as Barbara calls them, as they form the cornerstone for comprehending the subject matter of this book. The above topic will be further explored in the upcoming pages.

Now, these expansive topics will be addressed individually, and Barbara's teachings, tips, and lectures will be elucidated and summarized here. This will provide a comprehensive understanding of her perspectives on specific subjects. It's noteworthy that some of these topics are further subdivided into various areas.

Pure Air

Air is by far the most important thing in our lives; without it, we would not be able to survive. Every living human being is currently breathing air at this very moment; however, the majority of us could do more to attain better and purer air.

Oxygen is the most vital element in our life. Think of oxygen as the power for our tiny cell engines. Our cells need oxygen for energy, split into types: oxygen-dependent and oxygen-independent.

Clean air is vital for our well-being, ensuring our cells and body operate smoothly, providing us with more energy. When there's insufficient cellular oxygen, it can lead to hypoxia, causing symptoms like fatigue and headaches. Additionally, considering the impact of ions on air quality underscores the importance of natural environments, where negative ions dominate, creating a cleaner and more refreshing atmosphere. This underscores the essential link between breathing pure air and overall health.

Negative and positive ions

Ions are tiny particles in the air with different charges. They can freshen the air but may also cause changes when they interact. Negative ions, generated by movement, moisture, and air, are beneficial and abundant in natural settings like forests, waterfalls, and during thunderstorms. Negative ions are considered beneficial for fresh air.

On the other hand, positive ions, associated with a heavy atmosphere, are prevalent in urban areas due to pollution and lack of greenery. The air feels heavy if there are positive ions present. Positive ions in the air often signal an impending thunderstorm. Additionally, a crowded place with many people can contribute to a higher concentration of carbon dioxide being released.

Hence, the connection between ions and fresh air boils down to the prevalence of negative ions in natural spots, creating a cleaner and more refreshing environment.

Chronic Fatigue Syndrome and Oxygen Intake

Chronic fatigue syndrome is frequently associated with exposure to mold, which can impact our ability to take in oxygen. Mold can originate from diverse sources, including animals within the household and sleeping quarters. To safeguard optimal oxygen intake, it is advised to thoroughly investigate and uphold cleanliness in sleeping areas. Additionally, maintaining good posture and strengthening abdominal muscles plays a pivotal role in ensuring efficient breathing and optimal oxygen absorption. The emphasis on the importance of deep breathing, regular exercise, and preserving lung capacity underscores a holistic approach to well-being, acknowledging the interconnectedness of respiratory health and overall vitality.

Breathing at night

We do not have to consciously breathe during the night; in fact, our body does that automatically. However, we need to ensure we breathe the best possible air. The vast majority of people sleep with completely closed windows, and as a result, the air does not change, and we do not breathe in fresh air. This is one of the reasons why many people wake up feeling tired or exhausted. Slightly opening the window while we sleep contributes to making us breathe better air and waking up feeling more energized.

We understood thanks to Barbara's teachings that the quality of oxygen, the element that brings energy to our cell, is therefore key to breathing good oxygen.

Practical tips :

WHAT TO DO	BENEFITS
Open the Window slightly at night	You will wake up having breathed fresher air and with more energy.
Spending more time in nature	Cities are known to be more polluted, carrying more positive ions that have been explained to create 'heavy air,' which is worse for us.
Maintaining good posture during the day.	Maintaining good posture helps us breathe better by improving lung capacity and aligning respiratory muscles, making it easier to breathe effectively.
Stay away from mold	Clean the house, especially if animals live there, as they contribute to mold growth.
Exercise	Exercising promotes better and healthier lungs by enhancing oxygen intake.

Sunshine

Sunshine, the light from the sun, isn't just an incredible way to brighten our days; it's crucial for our health. It goes beyond lighting up our world; it plays a significant role in keeping our bodies in good shape by supporting various essential processes, as explained by Barbara. In this chapter, we'll delve deeper into this.

Barbara explained that it is necessary for our body to get at least 15 minutes of sunlight each day. Spending time in nature, especially in the morning with sunlight touching our skin has many benefits for our health :

- **Vitamin D Production :** Sunlight is a natural and primary source of vitamin D for our bodies. When our skin is exposed to sunlight's ultraviolet B (UVB) rays, it triggers the synthesis of vitamin D. This vitamin plays a crucial role in various bodily functions.

- **Calcium Absorption and Bone Health :** Vitamin D is incredibly important to help the absorption of calcium in the intestines. An efficient calcium absorption greatly contributes in maintaining robust bones and teeth. Preventing bone fractures and other problems.

- **Circadian Rhythm Regulation :** Exposing yourself to sunlight, especially in the morning, plays a role in regulating your body's internal clock, known as the circadian rhythm. This internal clock responds to daily patterns of light and darkness. When you're exposed to morning light, it sends a signal to your body that it's time to wake up and be alert.

  Therefore, seeing the sun improves the quality of your sleep at night. It contributes to a consistent and strong sleep-wake cycle, ultimately enhancing your overall sleep quality.

- **Influence on Hormonal Balance :** Sunlight has a direct impact on hormone production, like melatonin and serotonin. Serotonin levels increase when you expose yourself to morning light, which has a positive effect on your mood. Melatonin, the hormone that regulates sleep production, is closely linked to light exposure. Getting natural light during the day and allowing darkness in the evening supports the production of melatonin, which in turn helps kickstart and maintain a restful sleep.

Melonopsin

On top of what has been said so far, it is important to know that there is a receptor on the retina called "Melonopsin". This receptor is not involved in sight, but it is involved in brain function. Melonopsin absorbs blue lights. We know that the highest source of blue light is from the sun. Therefore, getting those blue lights from the sun through Melonopsin have several benefits:

- Tactical reasoning increase
- Ability to solve mathematical problems increased

These occurrences happen because the eyes are exposed to the sun. Of course, there's no need to stare directly at the sun, as that could be harmful to our eyesight. However, if you're outside on a sunny day and the sun is in your eyes, it is a normal and potentially beneficial experience.

Barbara also points out that individuals with darker skin tones may need more sun exposure. According to her studies, this is considered natural and straightforward, though it is often not discussed. She mentions that in America most of the population do not get enough sunlight during the day, due to various work commitments, lazy lifestyle and fear of getting skin cancer. Therefore, they do not get enough Vitamin D during the day and the calcium cannot get in and the minerals

Ultimately, it can be confidently stated that spending time in sunlight offers incredible benefits. Barbara suggests incorporating morning walks into our routine, allowing the sun to touch our skin. This practice not only enhances our overall well-being but also aligns with her recommendation for a healthier lifestyle.

Diet

Diet is arguably the topic of main importance in Barbara's teachings, or at least the one that is mentioned more often in her lectures and books, and therefore, it has vital importance. This chapter will scrutinize in depth her thoughts about diet and food.

To begin with, it is important to understand that Barbara advocates for a return to basic, natural, and whole foods. She gives significant importance to diet and suggests thinking about it thoroughly. She understands that the majority of people do not plan their meals thoroughly in advance, and that often leads to overeating and problems.

Barbara follows a plant-based, high-fiber diet rich in proteins. She consistently incorporates legumes into her meals. She primarily obtains her proteins from legumes, hummus, lentil burgers, marinated tofu, and incorporates nuts and seeds.
Fats are included in a controlled manner, primarily sourced from olive oil, with a teaspoon added to every meal. Additionally, she consumes nuts and seeds after each meal. Barbara mentioned that she has two meals per day. Her breakfast is her "Fruit meal," while her lunch is her "Vegetable meal," followed by an 18-hour fasting period.

As breakfast, she typically enjoys 2 or 3 pieces of fruit along with sourdough spelt toast drizzled with olive oil and topped with avocado. She compliments this with either red lentils, brown lentils, black-eyed beans, or scrambled organic tofu, accompanied by nuts and seeds. For lunch, it's usually a substantial salad, baked or stir-fried veggies, and legumes.

She rarely eats at night, and when she does, it is very light, like an avocado and a few crackers or a soup. Desserts are okay; she consumes them more or less once a week. She mentions having apple pie, which is made with spelt flour, and the apples are stewed. She adds sultanas or raisins. After baking the pie, she serves it with coconut cream or a nut cream.

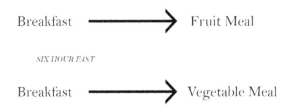

Barbara O'Neill makes a strong point about the importance of eating a consistent and balanced diet. She suggests that regularly choosing healthy foods is key to providing our bodies with the necessary nutrients. However, she mentions that it is very complicated to keep up with the news these days as there is uncertainty and not clear information about which food to eat, which food is okay and much information given are contrasting. Therefore, she aims with her studies to clarify the topic by giving her audience the best advice to follow a great diet.

Something that is vital in her teachings that she mentions often is that she strongly advises whole and unprocessed foods—natural and unaltered.

This consistent approach supports our overall health and well-being as nutrition directly shapes our overall well-being.

The mainstream research talks about food considering as the major players – carbohydrates, proteins, and fats. Claiming that our bodies require macronutrients for energy and essential bodily functions. In this chapter we'll delve deeper into this and we'll explore where to find these nutrients, their roles in your body, and the recommended proportions for maintaining a balanced diet. It is also vital to take into consideration micronutrients such as vitamins and minerals that play essential roles in maintaining health. Achieving the right balance is key to avoiding nutritional deficiencies.

Eating a balanced diet is vital for our well-being because it provides our bodies with the right mix of nutrients needed for optimal functioning. As explained by Barbara, the impact of our dietary choices extends beyond simply satisfying hunger; in fact, it affects :

- Energy levels
- Mental clarity
- The likelihood of developing conditions such as heart disease, diabetes, and obesity.

In a world full of diet trends always shifting, it's crucial to approach them wisely. Thanks to Barbara's teachings, in this chapter you will find tools to carefully evaluate nutrition information, to make informed choices that suit your specific individual needs.

Once you understand the basics, you can make smart choices that help your long-term health. Besides knowing about nutrition, finding peace in spiritual teachings can also make your mind feel calm and support a balanced body.

Barbara Food Pyramid

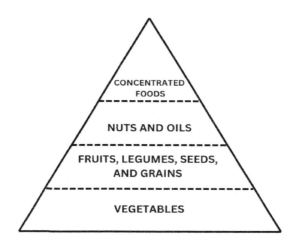

The new food triangle promoted by O'Neill is valued for its alkaline nature, protein content, fiber for the colon, cost-effectiveness, and availability. Vegetables, forming the base of the pyramid, are considered the most crucial element in our diet. Following that, other plant-based foods like fruits, legumes, seeds, and grains are included. Then, nuts and oil are recommended by Barbara for obtaining fats and proteins in our diet. Lastly, concentrated foods, which are nutrient-dense whole foods like fish, are emphasized.

Practical Tips :

→ Stop drinking with the meal.

→ Juice of a lemon with a tiny bit of boiling water just before the meal because the lemon is acid and it is a great digestive aid.

→ Frequent mixing of fruits and vegetables, if done daily, could compromise long-term digestive health. Therefore, she suggests avoiding it.

→ Follow the Barbara Food Pyramid to structure your meal planning.

pH Balance

What is the pH balance and why is it important?

pH balance is a measure to measure how acidic or alkaline something is. When acid is mixed with water, it releases hydrogen ions, while alkaline substances release hydroxide ions. The pH scale quantifies the concentration of these ions. A lower pH signifies more acidity, and a higher pH indicates more alkalinity. Maintaining a balanced pH level is crucial

<u>Acid alkaline Scale</u>

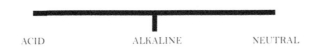

ACID   ALKALINE   NEUTRAL

The blood has a reading on the pH scale, that is between 7.3 and 7.4, if the pH scale goes up to 8 or 7.2, the person will go into a coma. We do not have to worry about the pH scale as there are two organs that keep it between that range: lungs and kidneys. However, it is important that we give our body the best food so that it works optimally.

Barbara employs the Hydrangea Analogy, where she compares the human body and a garden, emphasizing the profound impact of soil acidity or alkalinity on plant growth. In this analogy, our body's internal pH levels assume a crucial role in determining the health or disease of the "plant" (representing our body). Similar to how a garden's soil requires a specific pH range for optimal plant growth, our body's pH levels play a vital role in establishing an environment either conducive or resistant to cancer development. This analogy helps us comprehend the significance of maintaining a proper pH and being mindful of our dietary choices.

As you understood by the definition of pH balance, this topic introduces the concept of Alkalinity and Acid, which will be faced now.

Acid and Alkaline environment

Acid Environment:

The Acid environment in our body refers to things that are a bit more on the sour side. Like the stomach – it's naturally acidic for digesting food. But if our body gets too acidic for too long, it can mess up how things work inside us, possibly causing health problems.

The most common problems that eating acid-forming foods can create include chronic inflammation, digestive issues, joint pain, a weakened immune system, and potential impacts on bone health. If you find yourself experiencing one or more of these symptoms, Barbara's teachings become vital for you. More information about acid-forming foods will be provided shortly; for now, it is important to understand their potential effects. Barbara emphasizes that it's not necessary to completely eliminate acid-forming foods from our diet. Instead, striking a balance where most of our body is slightly alkaline is what keeps us feeling good and functioning well.

Alkaline Environment:

In our bodies, an alkaline environment means things are a bit on the basic side, helping our body work well. Having a pH level that's a bit on the alkaline side helps enzymes and cells in our body do their jobs right, which is good for our overall health. Our immune system works better in an alkaline environment.

Maintaining a slightly alkaline environment in the body acts as a strong defense against harmful bacteria and viruses. It helps lower the risk of inflammatory diseases by eliminating chronic inflammation associated with increased acidity, creating healing in our body. Keeping an alkaline balance contributes to robust bone health, preventing the loss of essential minerals.

Creating an alkaline environment in your body supports the process of getting rid of waste and toxins from your cells. Detoxification at the cellular level is a vital aspect of maintaining health. The human body works hard to keep a slightly alkaline pH because it's essential for many body functions. This balance is critical for making sure our cells work at their best, ensuring that the body's inner workings run smoothly.

How to create an Alkaline environment?

Most importantly, through a correct diet, as it will be shortly explained thoroughly. Moreover, stress, whether physically or emotionally, can make our body too acidic, causing a condition called acidosis. This excess acidity is not good for our health.

As suggested by Barbara, engaging in practices like meditation and deep breathing plays a role in pH regulation. It's about understanding that a calm and stress-free mind contributes to maintaining an internal alkaline state, fostering optimal well-being.

Therefore, aside from maintaining a correct diet, it is important to take care of our mental health as well. Barbara's teachings are extremely fascinating because they look at our body in a holistic view. Therefore, to make real changes and improvements, it is necessary to take care of several aspects of ourselves. There is no quick fix.

A good diet promotes alkalinity and can help alleviate the negative effects of persistent stress. It's like finding ways to bring our body back to a healthier balance during challenging times. Now, as promised, we'll delve deeper into the diet topic, exploring the Alkaline diet and the concepts of pH.

Alkaline diet - Applying pH Concepts to Health

In today's diet, packed with processed foods and too much sugar, our body's natural balance can get thrown off, leading to various health problems. The idea of giving preference to foods that promote alkalinity. It's like adjusting our diet to fit into a holistic approach for our overall well-being.

To create Alkaline conditions in the body it is necessary first of all to stay hydrated, which is crucial in this process. Drinking plenty of clean water aids our body's natural detox processes and keeps everything in balance. Water is right in the middle of the pH scale – it's neutral. By keeping ourselves well-hydrated, we're actually helping to create a balanced, slightly alkaline environment inside us which counteracts any acidic influences.

A key aspect of Barbara's teachings is the importance of using herbs in our diet to create an alkaline environment. In fact, she not only mentions their importance, but she believes they are necessary in everyone's diet. This chapter will soon explain what herbs she includes in her diet and suggests the most.

Eating foods that promote alkalinity is a key aspect of this holistic approach. Eating certain foods, which will be explained soon, can help you maintain a more alkaline diet. Understanding this can support your overall well-being.

Barbara shows us that to create Alkaline conditions through diet it is key in integrating alkaline-forming foods, such as fruits, vegetables, and legumes, into our daily meals. Consuming nutrient-rich foods packed with vitamins and minerals that help regulate the body's pH levels, helps to create an alkaline state. On the contrary, foods that lean towards acidity, like processed items and excessive animal products, can disturb this balance, potentially leading to various health issues.

Now let's list foods that are considered Alkaline forming foods by Barbara.

Alkaline-Forming Foods:

Alkaline foods	Notes
Lemon	It might seem counterintuitive as the lemon is acidic, but as explained by Barbara O`Neill, the Lemon is acidic for the only part of the body that should be acidic, which is the stomach. Without an acid stomach you cannot break the proteins down.

	When lemon is broken down in the gut and minerals dispersed, are dispersed into the blood and tissues it has an alkaline effect because the lemon is high in alkaline minerals which is sodium, potassium, calcium, magnesium and iron. These are the alkaline minerals.
Dark green leafy vegetables: Kale, parsley, collard greens, spinach, silverbeet kale.	Provide many minerals, have antioxidant properties, contribute to bone and heart health and have anti inflammatory effects.
Vegetables: baking sweet potato, pumpkin, and beetroot. (These three are just the most mentioned Dark green leafy vegetables, but Barbara includes more in her diet).	Vegetables have an alkaline effect. However, for some people it might have an acid effect. So, be careful of vegetables like: tomato, aubergine, and bell pepper.
Olive Oil	To fix the problem stated above it is suggested to prepare potato with olive oil as this makes the potato release a plant chemical, which is called "lycopene". Lycopene is from the fat soluble family. So, in simpler words we should be eating our meals with a bit of oil as it helps release the fat soluble vitamins. Lycopene is a very strong antioxidant and has the ability to reduce inflammation of the prostate gland.
Legumes. The most mentioned by Barbara are: Chickpeas, black-eyed beans, lima beans, lentils and soy.	Protein source, rich in fiber, contains phytoestrogens that contribute to hormonal balance especially in women, and contribute to stabilising blood sugar levels.
Millet and Quinoa	Barbara explains that millet and quinoa are usually part of the diet due to their incredible benefits. She suggests that these two foods need to be dressed, and some ideas suggested by Barbara O'Neill include using pear cream or lentils.
Almond and Brazil	Almonds are rich in proteins, vitamins, minerals and great for the heart. Brazil is rich in selenium, which is a mineral very important for having antioxidant properties and great for the immune system. It also has an anti-inflammatory effect.
Seeds	Seeds have anti-inflammatory antioxidant effects, as well as being a good source of Omega-3 and fiber. She normally consumes seeds after her breakfast as a source of healthy fats.
Savory Fruits	Tomatoes, avocados, lemons, eggplants, zucchinis, cucumbers, squash, pumpkin and aubergines. All of the above can be consumed as they offer

	some flexibility to our diet which plays a part in digestive health. However, if someone has a yeast presence in their boyd, eating a lot of fruit the sugar in the fruit would feed the yeast which would then give off acetic acid, lactic acid, uric acid
Herbs	Coriander and Turmeric are herbs that are advised by Barbara. They are all potent anti-inflammatory agents and are rich in vitamins and minerals.
Turmeric	Turmeric is known for its anti-inflammatory properties and beneficial effects on bone, digestive, and joint health, typically associated with alkaline-forming foods. However, Barbara advises caution due to potential irritants.
Ginger	Ginger is great for joint inflammation, both internally and externally (more on it later).
Potato	Potatoes are not only a source of vitamins and minerals but are also extremely useful, as explained by O'Neill, for fighting tissue inflammation.
Fresh cheeses like Feta or ricotta	Excellent sources of protein and calcium; moreover, they have a pH around 7, making them perfect for maintaining a balanced pH.
Natural Sweeteners: Maple syrup and Honey	They are natural sweeteners, making them great replacements for refined sugar. Moreover, they have antioxidant properties.
Healthy Fats	Go to page 43 for Fantastic Fats
Sourdough Bread (made from spelt or kamut)	Easier to digest than normal bread. It's nutrient-rich and has a lower glycemic index compared to normal bread.

Green vegetables are essential as they are a great source of magnesium. Barbara emphasizes the importance of magnesium, stating that it allows water to enter cells. Unfortunately, the majority of people in America either do not drink enough water or, for those who do, lack sufficient magnesium, making it challenging for water to penetrate cells.

Seeds are a great source of Omega-3 and this is one of the main reasons why they are so advised in our diet. Barbara emphasises the importance of including alpha-linolenic acid (ALA) in the diet, which is present in flaxseeds and chia seeds.

The foods mentioned above contribute to maintaining an alkaline environment in the body, which Barbara believes is essential for optimal health. She emphasizes the importance of a balanced diet with a focus on fresh, natural, and plant-centric foods. In the following pages, there will be a deeper research on some of the foods mentioned.

Benefits of living in an Alkaline Environment:

- Lower risk of inflammatory disease
- Contributes to robust bone health
- Immunes system works better
- Support cellular detox - eliminating waste and toxins from the cells
- Improve stress management

Acid-Forming Foods

These foods should be consumed in moderation or, in some cases, avoided. It's essential to include some acidic foods in our diet, but Barbara strongly advises against excessive intake of acid-forming foods for a healthy and well-functioning body. Barbara refers to "acid-forming foods" as those foods that create an acidic environment in our body.

Acid foods	Notes
Meat	Despite being a source of proteins and nutrients, Barbara suggests not consuming meat excessively and opting for natural meat instead of processed varieties. One issue that Barbara's studies highlight is the potential negative impact of excessive intake of saturated fats from meat.
Refined Sugar	It is common knowledge, and Barbara explains, that consuming refined sugar can have many negative effects. Among the numerous problems, the most common ones include obesity, diabetes, and inflammation. Barbara suggests opting for honey or maple syrup as alternatives.
Hybridized wheat	Barbara explains that changes made to wheat varieties, such as modifications through hybridization, can cause digestive problems or other health issues in certain individuals. Therefore, in alignment with her teachings, she advocates for eating whole and unprocessed foods as a key part of a balanced and health-conscious diet. This perspective emphasizes the idea that choosing ancient or unmodified grains could contribute to overall well-being.
Aged Cheese	As explained in O'Neill's studies, the blue in blue-vein cheese is mold. Therefore, she strongly recommends not consuming aged cheese. Just as it is crucial to keep the house clean to avoid mold, which can impact us and the air we breathe, we must be even more careful not to include it in our diet.
Caffeine	Caffeine has the potential to lower magnesium

	and calcium levels in the body, resulting in dehydration, heart irregularities, and disruptions in heart rhythms. Additionally, caffeine interferes with neurotransmitters, impacting the nervous system. Therefore, it is strongly advised to reduce excessive caffeine intake.
Alcohol	It is not food, but it creates an acid environment in the body. It is well-known to negatively impact our body, so this one is common knowledge. Therefore, Barbara suggests eliminating it from our lifestyle and diet.
Tobacco	As explained for alcohol, tobacco is another substance often consumed that creates an acidic environment in the body.
All the other legumes, grains and nuts apart from the one stated among the "alkaline foods"	It is strongly advised by Barbara not to consume legumes other than Lima beans, lentils, and soy. She also advises against eating grains other than millet and quinoa, and she recommends avoiding any nuts other than almonds and Brazil nuts. This is because they all create an acidic environment in our bodies.
Black Pepper	Black pepper is considered quite acidic, and Barbara suggests avoiding its consumption. In fact, she recommends coriander as a healthier alternative, as black pepper can potentially cause more problems for our digestive system and gut health.
Processed food	It is quite common knowledge, and Barbara insists on avoiding processed food. Processed food must be avoided at all times since consuming it, sadly common in our diet for many people, creates acidity in our body, leading to inflammation and diseases.

Foods high in phosphorus, sulfur, and chlorine are considered acidic. Consuming predominantly acidic foods has been associated with an increased prevalence and spread of conditions like cancer and heart disease. Therefore, it's crucial to maintain a balance, ensuring that the diet is predominantly alkaline as explained earlier. Although a small amount of acidity is needed for various bodily functions, moderation and a focus on alkaline-forming foods can contribute to overall health and well-being.

Water

Water is the second most vital element in our lives, following oxygen, which takes the top spot. Barbara ranks sodium as the third and potassium as the fourth most crucial elements. Seawater, rich in minerals, holds the highest concentration of sodium, constituting 92 minerals. From this, we derive common salt used in our daily lives, with 30% being sodium and 50% chloride.

Later on, there will be a section dedicated to salt, exploring its benefits and providing guidance on how to choose it.

Barbara emphasizes the essential role of water, she often says "We need water for every single movement and step".

She also explains that water is key and often underconsidered for relatively common problems such as headaches. She highlights its significance by noting that headaches, for instance, are common when we don't consume enough water.

Water is a vital player in maintaining the delicate balance of bodily functions, ensuring everything runs smoothly and you stay in good health.

Barbara explains that 2 liters of water is ideal to have it daily, reminding that fruits and vegetables contain water

Water at a cellular level

On a cellular level, water is crucial for facilitating essential biochemical reactions that keep our body functioning properly. It also plays a vital role in ensuring that nutrients reach their intended destinations, contributing to an overall sense of vitality and energy for both our bodies and ourselves.

Benefits of being hydrated

- **Water acts as a thermostat:** When our body gets warmer due to exercise or a hot day for example, we tend to sweat. This happens thanks to the water in our body. Sweating is a vital part of this natural process, helping maintain the perfect body temperature. By staying well-hydrated, these cooling mechanisms work effortlessly.

- **Detoxification processes:** The kidneys have the important role of filtering your blood to toxins making an exit via urine. This process heavily relies on water. Therefore, keeping hydrated is crucial to enable our body cleansing mechanisms. The kidney balances the sodium and water levels in the body, so it is an indication that the kidneys are not very happy when we have swollen legs. So, it is suggested to increase water intake and salt intake. There is the misconception that the water in the legs means we have too much water, and we should drink less. That is false. In fact, that only means that the water is not getting in the cells, but it is outside of the cells. We need magnesium for the water to get into the cell, Magnesium pulls the water into the cell.

- **Prevent injuries and improve joint health** : Water lubricates your joints, ensuring the movement happen smoothly. Barbara shows us how being hydrated reduces the risk of exercise-related injuries, important for anyone from elderly to athletes.

- **Enhances cognitive function and mood efficiency** : Dehydration impacts cognitive function and mood. Drinking water is incredibly important for optimal brain function

A deeper analyze on some food

Bread

Barbara talks about bread and how some bread is hard for tummies to digest. She says that long ago, people made special bread that was good for tummies. If we eat too much of the hard-to-digest bread, it can make our tummies feel funny. She tells us that some people today feel yucky because they eat too much of the hard-to-digest bread. Barbara suggests trying different foods that are good for our tummies.

Her studies go into detail about the complexities of bread. Unlike the mainstream focus on the benefits of fiber and B vitamins, she turns her attention to the starch structure. Specifically, she highlights amylopectin A, which she considers a bit of a troublemaker generated through the hybridization process. Amylopectin A causes disturbances in our body. However, ancient grains like spelt or kamut, managed to bypass the amylopectin A dilemma.

Therefore, O`neill strongly advised to consume bread with grains like spelt or kamut as a healthier and better choice for our system. Another option that Barbara mentions is a special way of making bread called "sourdough," which is easier for tummies. The fermentation process of this bread reduces the impact of amylopectin A.

Salt and Celtic Salt

Common table salt can be very harmful to us if consumed regularly and excessively due to its mineral composition. Barbara explains that the sodium chloride crystals are mixed with aluminium to produce table salt. Therefore, Barbara opted for a healthier option which is "Celtic salt", which contains 82 minerals. Celtic salt is a great source of magnesium, which aids in quick hydration. In fact, its significant magnesium content allows cells to pull water inside them rather than it being outside. This benefits cell health and their various essential functions in our body.
Barbara frequently emphasizes the benefits of Celtic Salt and encourages its consumption once or twice a day. The best way to consume Celtic Salt in one's diet is to place the salt on the tongue before drinking water, doing so helps our body retain minerals that we get rid of when we sweat or when we use the toilet. Alternatively, it can be used while cooking.

Sugar and Refined Sugar

Barbara explains that certain foods, like sugar, are incredibly good for plants but might not be ideal for us in excess. She discusses the impact of foods on our well-being, highlighting those that contribute to feeling good and others that may have less favorable effects. Barbara advocates for simplicity in our dietary choices, drawing a parallel to how our bodies, like flowers, respond with different "colors" to various foods. She emphasizes the importance of treating our bodies kindly and suggests sharing delicious and healthy foods with friends.

Sugar from fruits is beneficial for our health, but it should be consumed in moderation. Practicing moderation in sugar intake is a fundamental aspect of a healthy diet. On the other hand, refined sugar is to be absolutely avoided as it disrupts blood sugar levels and overall well-being. O'Neill understands that refined sugar is unfortunately very prevalent in today's diet. Therefore, she strongly emphasizes the importance of avoiding it and making mindful decisions when purchasing food, considering its genetically modified nature and its impact on blood sugar regulation.

Refined sugar can be found in various products, but Barbara specifically highlights three categories :

- Processed foods
- Candies
- Sodas

Barbara focuses on these three sources of refined sugar, pointing out the need to be vigilant about their presence in our diets.

Grains - Oatmeal and Rice

When discussing grains, numerous viewpoints exist, with various "experts" presenting entirely different theories on the topic. Thankfully, Barbara O'Neill's teachings provide valuable insights that challenge common beliefs about grains, revealing their inherent health benefits. O`Neill strongly advised to consume whole grains like unprocessed oatmeal. The less a product is processed, the better. She often talks about keeping our body on the Alkaline side for better health. Eating oatmeal and rice helps to make our body more alkaline, which is good for our health. Barbara challenges the idea that all grains make our body more acidic. She wants us to understand that our food choices can affect the balance in our body, and some grains, like oatmeal and rice, can make our body more alkaline and healthier.
Her thoughts on oatmeal and rice align with a broader philosophy of appreciating what nature gives us. This part discusses how, when we carefully choose these grains, we follow the principles of natural, unprocessed nutrition. Barbara's insights act as a guide for fostering a harmonious connection between individuals and the grains they include in their diet.

Oatmeal represents for many people a source of carbohydrates for sustained energy for breakfast, O`neill suggests trying it in other meals too as it is considered a versatile food. More importantly, oatmeal contains essential nutrients such as vitamins, minerals, and antioxidants, contributing to overall health.Oats contain a type of fiber called beta-glucans, which is soluble and known to have a positive effect on heart health by aiding in the reduction of cholesterol levels.

It is important not to store cooked rice at room temperature as it can easily grow mold and mycotoxins. Barbara explains that rice can develop mold or mycotoxins very quickly; she mentions a heart disease outbreak in Japan at the beginning of the 20th century caused by the mold present in stored cooked rice. Therefore, she strongly recommends eating cooked rice straight away or, as an alternative, storing it in the fridge and consuming it within no more than 24 hours.

However, when it comes to consuming food rich in carbohydrates, Barbara advises us not to exceed, as she advocates a non-carbohydrate-intensive diet. Therefore, it is suggested to consume small portions.

Legumes

Legumes are extremely important in our diet as sources of protein and high nutritional values that elevate our health and well-being. Plant-based proteins, like chickpeas, for instance, are essential contributors to a holistic diet. Among the most suggested legumes mentioned by O'Neill, with a high source of proteins, are:

- Chickpeas
- Black-Eyed Beans
- Kidney Beans
- Lentils
- Lima Beans

These legumes are not only high sources of proteins but also rich in fiber, which is important for gut health and sustaining energy levels throughout the day, among many other benefits. It is also necessary to point out something great about legumes: they are a crucial presence in our diet due to being a source of vitamins, minerals, and antioxidants. This makes them excellent for strengthening our immune system. Contrary to some mainstream beliefs that view these protein sources as inducing acidity, the legumes mentioned above play a role in the body's acid-alkaline balance, having alkaline potential.

Barbara suggests incorporating these legumes into various dishes, as their versatility makes them an appealing choice for different meals. In fact, following a diet that is good for our body does not have to be a chore; it can be a moment to express creativity in the kitchen, making the diet something to look forward to rather than a 'to-eat list'.

O'Neill often talks about ethical and sustainable practices, and eating legumes is in line with her view on environmental consciousness.

Anti-Inflammatory Foods

Anti-inflammatory foods are incredibly important to eat for anyone, regardless of gender, age, and fitness level. If someone practices sports, it is going to benefit them to eat anti-inflammatory foods to be able to practice and drastically reduce the chances of getting injured or experiencing chronic pain.

If someone is not doing much exercise, then it is arguably even more important, as eating the right food will improve not only their well-being. Opting for foods that support a balanced inflammatory reaction can be a positive contribution to overall health and well-being.

In line with O'Neill's holistic health beliefs, she advocates for eating specific foods, particularly those abundant in :

- Antioxidants
- Omega-3 Fatty Acids
- Anti-Inflammatory Components

Food rich in those contribute to reducing excessive inflammation. For this reason, whole foods like fruits, vegetables, nuts, seeds, and legumes are frequently emphasized for their ability to assist the body in handling inflammation as mentioned earlier.

This is the list of foods that have either antioxidant or anti-inflammatory effects :

Berries	Avocado	Olive Oil	Dark Chocolate
Leafy Greens	Salmon	Turmeric	Flax
Cruciferous Vegetables	Chia Seeds	Ginger	Brown rice and Quinoa
Fatty fish	Flaxseeds	Cayenne Pepper	Onion

Leafy greens

Leafy greens, in general, are renowned for their anti-inflammatory attributes, owing to their abundant supply of vitamins, minerals, antioxidants, and phytochemicals. Examples of Leafy Greens are:

- **Spinach :** Spinach is full of antioxidants, such as vitamins C and E, along with beta-carotene, which is great to fight inflammation.

- **Kale :** Kale has high levels of antioxidants, specifically flavonoids and carotenoids, known for their anti-inflammatory properties.

- **Arugula :** Arugula serves as a notable source of phytochemicals and antioxidants, contributing to its potential for anti-inflammatory effects.
- **Swiss Chard :** Swiss Chard, abundant in vitamins A and K alongside antioxidants, possesses anti-inflammatory properties.

Cruciferous vegetables

Cruciferous vegetables are well-known for their potential to reduce inflammation, thanks to their rich content of bioactive compounds such as antioxidants and anti-inflammatory phytochemicals. The most suggested cruciferous vegetables are :

- **Broccoli :** Broccoli has sulforaphane, which is a compound with anti-inflammatory and antioxidant properties.

- **Cabbage :** Cabbage offers a range of phytochemicals potentially contributing to its anti-inflammatory properties.

- **Cauliflower :** Cauliflower includes compounds like indole-3-carbinol, which has potential anti-inflammatory effects, and serves as a rich source of antioxidants.

Fatty Fish

Fatty fish are generally rich in Omega-3 fatty acids, contributing to heart health, joint health, eye health, and the fight against chronic inflammation. Among the fatty fish, those that are considered more anti-inflammatory include:

- **Salmon :** Salmon is rich in Omega-3, particularly in EPA and DHA, making it optimal for reducing inflammation and lowering blood pressure.

- **Mackerel :** Mackerel is also rich in Omega-3 and is considered the best among fatty fish for heart health.

- **Sardines :** Sardines are rich in Omega-3, considered a potent anti-inflammatory, and serve as a great source of Vitamin D and calcium.

Flax

Another important food is flax. Flax is highly suggested by Barbara as it is rich in Omega-3. It is important to consume freshly ground flax, or alternatively, if it is not ground fresh flax, then it should be kept in the freezer.

It is suggested keeping it in the freezer to preserve its nutritional value and prevent the degradation of essential fatty acids.

Cayenne Pepper

Cayenne pepper is frequently mentioned by Barbara O'Neill due to its numerous benefits. Firstly, it is rich in nutrients and is known for its cardiovascular advantages, helping to prevent heart attacks and strokes. According to Barbara's teachings, cayenne pepper is also considered beneficial for the thyroid gland.

However, it is advised not to consume cayenne pepper before bedtime as it can be stimulating. To ensure a peaceful night of sleep, it is recommended to avoid its intake before going to bed.

Cayenne Pepper benefits include :

- **Metabolism Boost** : Consuming cayenne pepper regularly improves metabolism, aids in burning calories, and its capsaicin makes you feel full, reducing the sense of appetite and assisting in weight management.

- **Pain Relief** : Cayenne pepper contains capsaicin, a natural pain reliever. It is beneficial for various situations, as Barbara mentions its effectiveness for arthritis, joint problems, and migraines.

- **Heart Health** : Cayenne pepper boosts heart health by preventing blood clot formation, clearing artery deposits, and improving circulation. It addresses issues like palpitations and arrhythmia.

- **Cancer Protection** : Barbara conducts studies suggesting that the plant chemicals in cayenne pepper, including capsaicin and flavonoids, may contribute to heart and cancer protection.

Barbara suggests incorporating cayenne pepper into dishes and gradually increasing its presence in our lives. She understands its benefits and emphasizes the importance of not overusing it, making it key to avoid excess intake.

However, it is advised not to consume cayenne pepper before bedtime as it can be stimulating. To ensure a peaceful night of sleep, it is recommended to avoid its intake before going to bed.

Charcoal

Charcoal is frequently highlighted in lectures for its remarkable capacity to draw and neutralize toxins and poisons. In instances of poisoning, hospitals present patients with the option of either stomach pumping or ingesting charcoal. If patients opt for charcoal, as suggested by Barbara, it is consumed with water. The ingestion of charcoal can bring relief from issues such as diarrhea, gastric discomfort, and bloating.

Charcoal, along with other elements and foods recommended by Barbara, can be utilized externally for various benefits. Creating a "Charcoal poultice" is simple and feasible, as charcoal effectively absorbs and combats toxins, providing pain relief. The poultice can be made by mixing charcoal with linseed or slippery elm.

The charcoal poultice is applied for :

- Insect bites, such as bee stings, spider bites, and snake bites
- Swelling
- Wounds
- Sore eyes

An advanced option surpassing traditional charcoal is activated charcoal, valued for its finely powdered consistency and increased potency. Activated charcoal undergoes a distinct preparation process, resulting in enhanced adsorption capabilities, making it particularly valuable for absorbing toxins, especially in medical scenarios for addressing poisonings and overdoses. Additionally, the purity of activated charcoal intended for consumption is another difference that makes it a more appealing choice compared to regular charcoal.

Onion

Onions have antioxidant and anti-inflammatory properties. Possessing both of these qualities makes them a highly recommended food in line with Barbara O'Neill's teachings.

Moreover, cutting an organic raw onion releases onion juice, which stimulates the respiratory organs and helps clear and clean the mucus. Cooked onions are beneficial for the ears, while raw onions are effective for respiratory issues. In addition to its typical use in meals, which offers numerous benefits due to its richness in nutrients, antioxidants, anti-inflammatory effects, and overall goodness for the heart and digestion, Barbara explains a unique way to use onions.

According to her, it is necessary to start by using a small and hygienic plastic bag. Place the onion in the plastic bag, then make the onion come in contact with your foot, and finally, put on a sock. It might seem strange, she says, but it has great value and benefits as it can cure a chest cold or head cold. The detailed explanation for why this happens will be provided in the upcoming chapter on "Natural Remedies."

Ketogenic Diet

The ketogenic diet, with its focus on healthy fats and less carbs, is suggested, especially for epilepsy. It suggests this diet might be good for the brain by offering a different kind of energy, as seen in the positive outcomes for people with epilepsy using excess coconut oil. While stressing the need for balanced fats from sources like nuts and seeds, the script indirectly ties the diet to better mental well-being by connecting its benefits to overall brain function. But, it's important to know that the script lacks detailed proof or talks about possible downsides of the ketogenic diet. It signals that more research and expert advice are needed for a full picture.

The Ketogenic Diet is known for its potential benefits and its impact on neurological health. Ketones, produced when the body breaks down fats, show promise in healing and protecting the brain.

Coconut Ketogenic Diet

The Ketogenic diet can have a slightly different variation in a diet called "Coconut Ketogenic Diet" it consists in :

- Dropping the carbohydrates

- Eat high fiber
- Generous proteins
- Healthy fats

The healthy fats she suggests are nuts, seeds, olive oil and coconut oil. It is suggested to start with a teaspoon of coconut oil three times a day, building up to 4 teaspoons of coconut oil three times a day. The diet includes vegetables, especially legumes.

The Coconut Ketogenic diet is considered easier to eat and follow.

Fantastic Fats

The mainstream guidelines view consuming fat as an enemy, while it is an essential nutrient. Unfortunately there are many misconceptions with fats. In fact, many Americans who are obese and want to lose weight tend to listen to the media hype which encourages them to eat less fat as "fat makes you fat", therefore they are on a high carbohydrate diet. However, this is incorrect as fat gives you a sensation of satiation, which makes you stop eating. If you do not have fats you tend to overeat. Obviously, there are different types of fats. Some fats, especially processed ones are not good, but others are not only good but essential for having a healthy body and have benefits in weight loss too.

Barbara O'Neill emphasizes the importance of understanding the molecular structure of fats to comprehend their effects on the body and knowing what to eat. Fats divide in two main categories: saturated and unsaturated.

Saturated fats are often found in animal products and certain plant oils. Some fats are at first unsaturated and through a process they become saturated by adding hydrogen ions. The resulting saturated fat lacks the natural molecular structure found in unsaturated fats. It can not be naturally unsaturated and may have adverse effects on the body due to the unnatural structure. An example is Margarine.

She emphasizes the importance of consuming healthy, unaltered polyunsaturated fats like salmon, mackerel, flaxseeds, chia seeds, hemp seeds, nuts, and coconut oil. She also suggests eating unaltered monostaruated fats like avocado, some nuts, olive oil and dark chocolate. The discussion implies that the unnatural molecular structures of saturated and hydrogenated fats may not be well-processed by the body. Heart disease and skin cancer rates are mentioned to have risen with the introduction of margarine.

Being rich in medium-chain fatty acids, coconut oil stands out as an excellent source of energy. Notably, it doesn't necessitate bile or pancreatic lipase for digestion, allowing it to be absorbed directly into the bloodstream, providing a rapid energy boost. Furthermore, the oil is rich with antimicrobial properties and contains lauric acid, contributing to various health benefits, including weight loss. This reinforces Barbara's perspective that eliminating fats for weight loss isn't a wise decision. She emphasizes opting for the right fats, which she calls "Fantastic fats."

Our bodies rely on Essential Fatty Acids (EFAs) for optimal health since we can't produce them ourselves. Therefore, it is necessary to include food that has them in our diet, like :

- Flaxseed

- Coconut oil

In terms of Omega-3, the alpha-linolenic acid (ALA) found in flaxseed transforms into eicosapentaenoic acid (EPA) and docosahexaenoic acid (DHA) in our bodies. DHA, mainly found in fish, plays a crucial role in cell membrane function and repair.

Barbara O'Neill suggests being thoughtful in choosing fats, highlighting the importance of going for natural, unprocessed sources for overall health. It's a smart approach to well-being through mindful dietary choices. Barbara really stresses the idea of getting polyunsaturated fats from whole foods such as seeds and nuts instead of using extracted oils. She's suggesting a different way to look at our food intake, like a food pyramid but in the shape of a triangle. So, at the very bottom, we have vegetables, emphasizing how crucial they are. Then come fruits, legumes, and seeds, followed by grains. And right at the top, you've got nuts, oils, and concentrated foods. It's like a guide to encourage a diet where plant-based foods form the foundation, and more processed or concentrated items are kept in moderation.

Detox

"One of the best ways to detox is to stop eating for a couple of days. When we stop eating, all that energy that usually goes to digestion now starts to cleanse and detox through the body." This is one of the sentences said by Barbara that shows the importance of detox very simply in a few words. Obviously, the detox from eating for two days should not be done regularly, but it is a rare occasion that helps.

Detoxification stands as a cornerstone of maintaining overall well-being, focusing on the body's innate ability to eliminate toxins and support vital organs, particularly the liver. Barbara O'Neill talks about the crucial role of detoxification, getting more and more important in a world that is becoming more and more polluted. Detoxification does not only help our body but also improves our mental health and emotional aspects.

Cleansing is essentially the process of eliminating impurities and toxins from the body. It can be seen as a reset.

How to do a Detox?

Fasting can facilitate detoxification by enabling the body to redirect energy towards cleansing processes. In fact, health retreats conducted by Barbara O`Neill follow a structured detox program involving fasting, juices, and nutrient-rich meals.

Fasting, according to Barbara O'Neill, is essentially choosing not to eat for a while. This gives your body the chance to focus its energy on cleaning up, aiding in detox, and boosting your overall health. As stated earlier, O'Neill normally eats twice a day in a 6-hour window, followed by 18 hours without eating.

However, it is recommended to visit a doctor before making any decisions as everyone's needs and physical abilities are different. Barbara stresses the potential risks of doing long water fasts and highlights the importance of taking a balanced approach to detoxification. She emphasizes the need for protein intake, especially in the second phase of the detox process, as amino acids play a crucial role in neutralizing toxic metabolites.

Detoxification And Cleansing

When talking about detoxification and cleansing, she covers three main aspects :

- Difference between raw and cooked food
- The significance of minerals
- Creation of an alkaline environment
- The importane of liver

Raw vs Cooked Food

Due to the richness in enzymes and vital nutrients for our body, Barbara strongly advises including raw food in our diet. The vital nutrients are incredibly important for the process of detoxification and cleansing. If we go to a complete detox for two days, consuming exclusively juices then it is suggested that a gradual reintroduction of solid food begins with a 50/50 mix of raw and cooked foods.

The significance of minerals

Barbara emphasizes how important minerals are for detoxification, pointing out their crucial role in body functions. Minerals are needed for :

- Enzymes
- Cellular communication
- Getting rid of toxins

Adding minerals to your diet, along with eating raw foods, helps with detox and keeps you healthy overall.

Creation of an alkaline environment

The benefits of an alkaline environment and how to create one have already been thoroughly explained earlier. If you would like to know more about it, I encourage you to reread that chapter.

The importance of liver

The liver plays a crucial role in processing environmental toxins and managing glucose from carbohydrates. It is necessary to look after our liver as an excess of fructose, often found in sweetened foods can cause a Fatty liver, which can lead to more serious liver conditions. The detox process aims to support the liver in eliminating environmental toxins and promoting overall well-being.

The three phases of the liver detox are :

- **Phase one :** In this phase, the liver breaks down fat-soluble toxins into metabolites. During this phase of the liver detoxification process, antioxidants take center stage in supporting the liver's function. Antioxidants such as beta-carotene and vitamin C protect cells by giving electrons to neutralize harmful free radicals, reducing stress and keeping cellular structures safe. Minerals and B vitamins are also extremely important during detoxification. Together, they all collaborate to guide the liver through Phase One, ensuring the safe breakdown of fat-soluble toxins.

- **Phase two :** The liver combines these metabolites with amino acids to create a water-soluble state.

- **Phase Three :** The water-soluble toxins are released from the body through sweat glands, the colon, and the kidneys.

Barbara O'Neill underscores the importance of incorporating bitter liver herbs to rejuvenate liver function. The most recommended bitter herbs for the liver are:

- **Dandelion :** Dandelion is promoted for its role in supporting liver health. This herb is known also for its bitterness. Due to the bitterness, it might be challenging for some people directly. However, Barbara O`neill encourages direct consumption if possible.

- **Milk Thistle (Mary's Thistle) :** Another element often mentioned by O`neill due to its effectiveness in assisting the liver. Its bitterness is considered necessary and crucial for its benefits.

- **Gentian :** Gentian root can be taken as a supplement. That is probably the best way to consume them.

- **Ginger :** Due to its potential benefits for digestion and liver health, ginger is considered an herb recommended for the liver.

- **Lemon :** As also mentioned before, the lemon has alkaline properties in the tissues. Lemons are renowned for their detoxifying effects and overall health support.

Due to the difficulty of consuming some of those products due to their taste, especially their bitterness, Barbara mentions that these herbs can be taken as capsules or tablets as they can still enjoy their benefits without directly experiencing the pronounced bitterness.

It's crucial to note that the emphasis on bitter herbs aligns with traditional herbal medicine and holistic teachings. The bitter taste is believed to stimulate digestive juices and facilitate the liver's detoxification process, enhancing digestive processes and contributing to overall well-being.

Benefits of Detoxification and Cleansing

- **Enhanced overall health** : Getting rid of toxins through detox helps improve overall health by supporting vital organs and creating a balanced internal environment. It boosts the body's ability to work at its best and keeps us feeling good.

- **Cellular restoration** : Detox aids cellular restoration and renewal. This allows the body to repair damaged cells.

- **Potential longevity** : Detoxification, by removing harmful substances and promoting cellular health, is thought to contribute to potential longevity as a cleaner internal environment lower the risk of diseases and strengthen the body.

- **Weight management** : Proper detox programs help in weight management by encouraging the breakdown of fat stores. It is important to understand that detox is a serious program, and detox does not mean "I eat less or I do not eat at all to lose weight". It should be a conscious and intelligent choice, preferably made with the help of a specialist, that among several benefits brings this one too.

- **Improved digestion** : During detox, the process of digestion does not happen, enabling the body to channel energy into cleaning and healing. This break can enhance digestion, as the digestive system gets a rest, and the body focuses on getting rid of waste and rejuvenating itself.

To sum it up, "Detoxification" is a big part of staying healthy in a holistic way – it's like giving our body a fresh start. Picking foods that help balance things inside and following detox plans goes along with the idea of making our insides more alkaline. This helps the body get rid of acidic waste, keeping us full of life and healthy. Just remember, these are tips and suggestions from Barbara. But, adjustments are made based on each person's health and what they like.

Sleep

Sleeping is something that everybody does, and it is incredibly important for so many reasons. However, it is often not given enough importance. It is not just about quantity, but the quality that makes the difference, as Barbara says.

Before starting to talk about it, it's important to mention that Barbara, in her lectures, often references the book "Why We Sleep?" by Matthew Walker, bringing insights from the book into her teachings.

Why is sleeping important?

What happens if we don't sleep or sleep not much? O'Neill explains that if we do not get enough sleep, something happens. In the prefrontal cortex, it forms amyloid plaques, which can cause Alzheimer's or severe dementia. Barbara mentions famous people like Margaret Thatcher and Ronald Reagan who went on with 5 hours of sleep and ended up having severe dementia. Therefore, to avoid amyloid plaques, we need to sleep.

The benefits of sleeping are the following :

Benefits	Notes
Physical Health	Sleeping helps the rejuvenation of the cells, and tissues as well as strengthening the immune system.
Mental Health	It improves mood, preventing mood swings. Barbara mentions that often people get upset about something because they have not eaten well or slept enough.
Cognitive Function	Sleeping is the vital key to learning and improving memory, as well as concentration and focus. Also, sleeping works as a cleaning system for the little calcified deposits that might begin. Preventing Alzheimer's or dementia.
Metabolic Health	Lack of sleep is connected to effects on appetite and metabolism, causing the individual to overeat.
Cardiovascular Health	High-quality, consistent sleep contributes to a lower risk of cardiovascular diseases.
Overall Well-being	Increased energy levels and vitality.

Individual sleep needs may vary, but consistently prioritizing sufficient and quality sleep is fundamental for overall health and well-being.

How to maximize your sleep quality?

Barbara's advice is not extensive, but it is extremely important and might sound unfamiliar to the majority of people. Several factors contribute to poor sleep quality:

- **Lack of Exercise :** Lack of exercise contributes to poor sleep. Insufficient physical activity during the day can negatively impact sleep. Regular exercise is mentioned as a factor that enhances sleep quality.

- **Dehydration :** Not drinking enough fluids has a negative effect on sleep. Having drank a sufficient amount of water per day, Barbara suggests 2L, is essential for a good night's sleep.

- **Late Nights :** Sleeping late has a very negative impact on memory consolidation. Going to bed late is associated with hindering memory consolidation. The text suggests that individuals who go to bed at midnight might experience challenges with their short-term memory unit, affecting overall memory. Going to sleep at midnight means that melatonin is cut in half. Additionally, you can wake up the following day and have short-term memory from the day before. There have been research studies conducted by Matthew Walker, who, for instance, took 20 students – 10 of whom slept 6 hours and 10 who had 8 hours of sleep. The second group retained almost double compared to the first group of the things they studied during the day.

- **Large Late Meals :** Barbara explains that sleeping with a full stomach, especially after a large late meal, can hinder the rest of the stomach. This is linked to the idea that the stomach needs a break during sleep, and having a big meal late at night could disrupt this process. O`Neill does not have dinner and if she has, she tends to have an extremely light meal.
- **Technology in the Bedroom :** In her lectures she mentioned several times that one of the common reasons why these days people do not sleep well is due to the negative impact of technology in the bedroom, particularly the electromagnetic fields from devices. Using technology, especially looking closely at devices like smartphone, laptop or television can disrupt sleep, and the prevalence of technology in bedrooms is identified as a contributor to insomnia.

- **Bad Air in the Bedroom :** It is strongly advised that the window is kept slightly opened at night guaranteeing that you breathe good air, so that you sleep better and wake up feeling more refreshed. Moreover, the impact of moldy pillows as well as inadequate ventilation, can affect sleep.

- **Sunshine :** Seeing the sunshine, especially during the morning, is extremely important as it aligns the body with natural circadian rhythms. This practice is often neglected by individuals who do not spend enough time in the sunshine, and it can disrupt sleep.

All the above factors emphasize the significance of addressing different lifestyle and environmental aspects to improve sleep hygiene and overall well-being. It is not one action that creates great results for better sleep, but it is the togetherness of small actions that makes an extraordinary difference. Another piece of advice given by Barbara is to take a hot shower or bath before bedtime, possibly with Epsom salts or lavender essential oil, as a way to enhance sleep.

The importance of Early Nights and Screens Off :

Above, the importance of going to sleep early and avoiding screen use before bedtime has been mentioned. Now, we'll delve deeper into these two key points. O'Neill emphasizes their significance for overall well-being, as neglecting them can lead to various complications. Adhering to these rules:

- **Going to sleep early :** Ideally, at 10 pm in summer and 9 pm in winter, is not merely about physical repair but also about mental rejuvenation.

- **Quit technology before bed :** Artificial light interferes with your body's natural rhythm, disrupting the essential sleep you need.

While we sleep, there is a tiny gland in the base of our brain called "The pineal Gland" that releases four hormones every night, between 10 pm and 3 am. In the winter it is between 9 pm and 2 am. What are those:

- **Serotonin :** The mood hormone. To increase the production of this hormone it is also suggested to keep a cheerful and happy disposition and laugh a lot. Simply being happy and finding the positives in every situation helps the increase of this hormone.

- **Melatonin :** The hormone that fixes and rejuvenates during the nighttime. Like for serotonin, laughing and being happy increase the production of this hormone.

- **Arginine Vasotocin :** A hormone that puts you in a deep sleep

- **Epithalamion :** A hormone that increases learning capacity and slows down aging

Practices like fasting and sleeping in darkness help to enhance hormone production, in opposition to caffeine, alcohol, and excessive meat consumption, which can inhibit it. Recognizing the importance of an early bedtime and avoiding screens is key for ensuring a deep and restorative sleep, allowing the body to maximize the release of essential hormones.

Sleep cycles

Between 10 PM and 3 AM, there is a significant hormonal activity of various processes aiming to do different functions in our body. Therefore, our body is meant to be sleeping at that time. Barbara insists on going to sleep early, by 10 pm. Sleep should be treated and regarded as a scheduled appointment that demands respect. However, with the current lifestyles that many people lead, adhering to this practice is becoming increasingly challenging.

The concept of sleep cycles is interesting to understand even more why going to sleep early is important and what happens while we sleep. First of all, it is necessary to know that nighttime sleep is divided into cycles that differ from each other and are essential for various physiological and cognitive functions. Before delving deeper into timings and cycles, it is necessary to know that sleep can be divided into two types of sleep cycle : NREM and REM.

REM (Rapid Eye Movement) sleep is when we dream a lot, our eyes move quickly, and our muscles stay still. NREM (Non-Rapid Eye Movement) sleep starts with lighter stages (1 and 2) and then goes into deep sleep (Stage 3). This deep sleep, also known as slow-wave sleep (SWS), is super important for our body to heal and grow because it has slow brain waves.

To sum it up and simplify it, it can be said that REM is for dreaming, and NREM, especially Stage 3, is for deep and restorative sleep.

These are the sleep cycles :

- **9 PM to 10:30 PM :** 80% NREM and 20% REM.

During the early part of the night, most of the sleep is focused on NREM (Non-Rapid Eye Movement), which includes stages crucial for memory consolidation and bodily restoration, which is key for learning and recovery.

- **10:30 PM to 12 AM :** 60% REM, 40% NREM.

As the night progresses, there's a shift toward a higher percentage of REM (Rapid Eye Movement) sleep, linked to vivid dreaming and memory consolidation. However, NREM (Non-Rapid Eye Movement) continues to play a significant role throughout the sleep cycle.

- **12 AM to 1:30 AM :** 50/50 ratio between NREM and REM.

An equal distribution suggests a balance between the stages, potentially contributing to overall sleep quality.

- **1:30 AM to 3 AM :** 40% NREM, 60% REM.

A shift towards a higher proportion of REM sleep underscores the significance of dreaming and memory processing during this period.

- **3 AM to 5 AM :** 20% NREM, 80% REM.

The late-night hours are characterized by a dominance of REM sleep, potentially involving intensified dreaming and additional memory consolidation.

Sleep cycles show how sleep is dynamic, helping with many things like memory, learning, and emotions. Going to sleep early helps as it is natural for our body to go through the cycle as it is supposed to be. Getting a full night's sleep is key for both NREM and REM stages, supporting cognitive and physical well-being.

Follow this summarized set of practical tips for improved sleep :

- → Avoid screens before going to sleep.
- → Air your room during the day, and keep the window open overnight for better sleep.
- → Establish a routine of going to bed early.
- → Get sunlight during the day, especially in the morning. Barbara explains that the darker your skin, the more sunlight you need.
- → Avoid caffeine, stimulants, and herbs like Cayenne pepper.
- → Exercise daily.

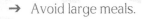

→ Avoid large meals.

Exercise

The value and benefits of exercising go beyond simply being fit and performing simple physical activity. It is necessary for overall well-being. It represents a valuable investment in one's health, bringing benefits across various aspects of life. This section explores the profound impact of exercise, highlighting its dynamic role in shaping the body, mind, and overall vitality.

Daily exercise is great for cognitive function, and reduces the risk of neurodegenerative diseases.

Barabara often says that regular exercise is excellent for warming the blood and enhancing circulation. It's crucial to prevent cold feet, indicating poor circulation, and exercise plays a key role in maintaining warmth and circulation.

Burning calories and building muscles

Exercise serves as a metabolic investment, burning calories and promoting weight management. Moreover, exercising is a way to build, strengthen, and maintain them. From resistance training to endurance exercises, you enhance the muscular currency that supports daily activities, from lifting groceries to maintaining posture.

It has benefits for bones too as regular training ensures strong and resilient bones. Studies conducted by Barbara showed how exercising prevents osteoporosis and improves bone density.

The last well-known physical benefit that exercise brings is the reinforcement of the immune system, reducing susceptibility to illnesses. It leads to fewer sick days and overall health resilience.

Muscle know no age

Barbara emphasizes in her teachings that "Muscles know no age," implying that regardless of your age, you can maintain a healthy and fit body. It's crucial to prepare for later years by providing the body with ample water, nutritious food, and, equally important, regular exercise. While some claim to be too busy for exercise, Barbara explains the existence of a type of workout that only takes 15 minutes a day yet yields magical benefits. For those with physically demanding jobs like Personal Trainers, Barbara suggests that's already beneficial. However, for the majority neglecting exercise, she believes that daily physical activity has the potential to transform lives.

What is the "secret" exercise?

Barbara claims that the best training for better health is HIIT (High-Intensity Interval Training). This training involves short bursts of intense activity followed by recovery: 20 seconds of work, 60 seconds of recovery, repeated 6 times. The timings can vary, with some trainers suggesting 30 seconds of training and 90 seconds of recovery for 6 cycles. HIIT can be performed on a bike, while running, or during swimming. Research suggests staying active during recovery; gentle stretching or slow walking is highly recommended. Perform the exercises at a slow pace. The recovery time serves as an indicator of fitness – the more you need it, the less fit you are. The encouraging news is that consistent exercise will lead to improvement. In essence, HIIT is a water activity that elevates your heart rate and breathing.

When to exercise?

Exercising must be done every day. Exercising in the morning has incredible health benefits, as a network of capillaries is opened that equals the distance around the planet earth (hard to believe, I know). These capillaries are in the extremities of our body, therefore it have a lot of health benefits:

Health Benefits
Lymphatic System Activation
Cell Strengthening
Bone and Muscle Strength
Balance Improvement
Vision Enhancement
Warmer Body
Mental and emotional benefits
Increased circulation

HIIT, as you understand, is crucial if you want to have a healthy and long life. Studies show that by the age of 50, the majority of people lose 40% of their lung capacity. This happens because, as people age, it is common to decrease the amount of exercise and never experience the sensation of "increased breathing" and the body telling you "This is enough," but you keep going. Going beyond your mental limit to experience the struggle that leads to increased breathing is a life-changing experience. It might not be pleasant at the moment, but it has enormous benefits.

Earlier in the book, it was mentioned how oxygen is the most vital element of our life. Therefore, you should understand how ensuring our lungs are capable of getting 100% oxygen is key.

What happens in our body?

You already know the benefits; however, let's delve into what happens internally. At the end of your first burst of intense activity, the body taps into the glycogen stores. By the end of the second set, the glycogen stores are depleted, but the body needs fuel. Therefore, the body triggers a release of the Human Growth Hormone.

This hormone works until we reach a certain age and naturally stop growing; then, the hormone goes into retirement. When we engage in HIIT, that hormone is brought out of retirement. This hormone induces the release of "Hormone-Sensitive Lipase," an enzyme that breaks down fat cells – the body's fuel store. Glucose burns in the body at 4 calories per gram, while fat burns at 9 calories per gram. Therefore, fat provides more than double the energy that glucose does. So, fat is an excellent fuel for our body. Once this hormone is released, the body starts burning fat as fuel. As the hormone-sensitive lipase is activated, the switch occurs.

The most powerful form of exercise : Rebounding

It has been studied that HIIT is a wonderful way of exercising and can be done in many different ways. One form of exercise is known to be the most powerful, which is "Rebounding".

Rebounding (Jumping on a Mini Trampoline) :

Rebounding involves jumping on a mini trampoline, creating a bouncing motion.

Health Benefits :

- **Strength increased :** To increase strength you have got to define gravity, like for any strength exercise and rebounding enable do train that.

- **Lymphatic System Activation :** Rebounding is highly effective in activating the lymphatic system, acting as the body's vacuum cleaner to eliminate waste from tissues. The rebounder is effectively your 'lymphatic stimulator.' Our body has the heart, which is our pump to circulate blood everywhere. The lymphatic system does not have a pump. The lymphatic system is like a network of canals with gates. When we wake up in the morning, these gates are shut. When using the rebounder, as we jump and reach high points, the gates open; when we come down, the gates close. This activates the lymphatic system. A couple of minutes on the rebounder gets the lymphatic system activated for the whole day.

- **Cell Strengthening :** The bouncing motion provides a shock to every cell in the body, leading to overall cell strengthening. The constant acceleration and declaration shocks and challenges the cells in the whole body, strengthening them.

- **Bone and Muscle Strength :** Rebounding is a weight-bearing exercise, benefiting bone density and muscle strength.

- **Balance Improvement :** Regular rebounding helps reset mechanisms related to balance, making it an ideal exercise for those with balance issues.

- **Vision Enhancement :** Rebounding can contribute to strengthening eyesight through constant focus changes during the activity.

- **Cleansing tissues :** rebounding daily helps the body cleansing tissues

- **Remedy for Varicose veins :** Arteries carry oxygenated blood from the heart to the body, providing it with nutrients and oxygen. On the other hand, veins return deoxygenated blood from the body back to the heart. Therefore, Rebounding is successful in avoiding stuff like varicose veins. As on the rebounder we push those blood back to the top by stimulating calves.

Compared to other exercises, rebounding is unique in its ability to defy gravity, involving acceleration, deceleration, and constant shock to cells. In contrast to exercises with jarring impact, rebounding provides a safer option, making it suitable for individuals with knee, ankle, and hip problems. To understand the effectiveness of rebounding, it is important to know that NASA recognizes it as the only exercise increasing the g-force for astronauts, helping them handle the effects of space travel. It has been found to be effective in reducing muscle and bone loss experienced by astronauts in space. Practicing rebounding is described as a simple yet powerful exercise that can be easily incorporated into daily routines. It is accessible to various age groups and fitness levels, making it a versatile form of physical activity. It does not take much time and does not require much space.

Tips:

Regular rebounding for at least two minutes a day is recommended to activate the lymphatic system effectively. Simply a minute a day every hour is extremely useful if possible or 15 minutes consecutively during the day. There is no need to do lots of jumps. Simply a "health bounce" that is easy and somewhat relaxing to do while stimulating the body. It is presented as a fun and engaging way to maintain overall health, especially for those with limited time for exercise.

In summary, rebounding is portrayed as a highly accessible, enjoyable, and beneficial form of exercise, providing advantages for the lymphatic system, cellular strength, bone density, balance, and vision.

Human Growth Hormone (HGH)

The Human Growth Hormone (HGH) is crucial in our body, and sometimes there is the misconception that it is only important until around the late teenage years of our life. This is very incorrect, and we'll look deeper into it.

It is common knowledge that Human Growth Hormone (HGH) naturally comes into play during growth phases, especially in the teenage years, affecting things like height and overall development. During challenging times, HGH acts like an emergency responder in the body. In fact, at the time when we grow in height, our bones and structure change constantly.

However, HGH works later on in life too, especially in scenarios of prolonged stress, which is pretty common in adulthood nowadays. As the body perceives the stress as a threat, HGH functions as if it's sending out an emergency signal, gathering resources to deal with the stress. In simple terms, HGH acts as a versatile regulator, adjusting the body's responses to demanding circumstances.

Also, HGH enhances the body's ability to get the most from proteins in our food. At the same time, HGH is portrayed as a balancer of circulation, affecting blood flow to the skin, which could slow down aging. This connection shows how activating HGH can impact overall well-being. So, not only does the Human Growth Hormone help get the most from proteins, but it also has the effect of slowing down aging. Barbara explains that HGH might be the most underrated and unders-considered hormone. It is common knowledge that many people want to look younger and feel good, and HGH contributes to both.

How to increase the release of this hormone?

Now that you understand its importance, you are probably wondering how to benefit from it. Barbara explains that High-Intensity Interval Training (HIIT) is extremely useful and effective in waking up HGH's potential. HIIT, where you switch between intense activity and rest, is recommended to get HGH going. This exercise creates a sort of "mini-crisis" in the body, keeping HGH active for a remarkable 24 hours. The talk cleverly connects the dots, showing how a specific kind of exercise can work hand in hand with our hormones.

HGH increases circulation of the blood to the skin; the effect of this is that it slows down aging. It is known that there are several models of Hollywood actors and actresses who pay roughly 1000 dollars a week to get HGH, as looking good is key for their profession. Through 15 minutes a day of HIIT, you can get the same results. Moreover, once we do HIIT, the HGH remains active for 24 hours. Quality nuts, seeds, avocados, olive oils, and exercising every morning make you not miss out on HGH. Those foods have some specific nutrients that can influence HGH production.

To simplify graphically the role of HGH, we can Imagine HGH (Human Growth Hormone) as a messenger in our body. When it gets released, it sends a message to our body to break down stored fat. It's like a signal that helps our body switch from using sugar to burning fat more efficiently. This whole process is how our body manages weight by making good use of its energy sources. Therefore, HGH (Human Growth Hormone) can be seen as a helpful guide in our body, making sure our body uses protein from our food well, like a smart assistant. So, when we activate HGH, it's like giving our body a boost for overall well-being.

Mental Health

Barbara often talks about mental health and the importance of our brain. Our mental health is a fascinating topic and is very extensive, linked with many others like diet, exercise, sleep, and many more. In this chapter, we will try to cover Barbara's teachings, hoping to help you get these precious pieces of information.

First of all, mental health is a key part of the holistic approach that O'Neill uses, which necessarily means considering various lifestyle factors. The most mentioned are:

- Diet
- Sleep
- Physical activity
- Stress management

Diet

By now, you should know what is good and what's not good for our body. The earlier chapter about diet should have given you enough information to know what the best choices are to make. In fact, Barbara's teachings, as explained in the introduction, aim to give you the tools to make your own decisions, knowing more about how our body reacts to certain foods and in which environment we thrive. Consideration of the Ketogenic Diet, being rich in healthy fats, proves supportive of brain health, so it could be taken into consideration by certain individuals (see more on the page dedicated to the Ketogenic Diet earlier). Avoiding tobacco and alcohol is obviously very important for optimal brain function.

Sleep

There is a whole chapter about sleep, which is a cornerstone for mental well-being. Insufficient sleep not only affects cognitive function but also doubles the risk of mental illness.
Avoiding excessive electromagnetic fields before sleeping and during the day is also vital.
For Barbara, quality sleep underscores its non-negotiable role in mental well-being. The revelation that ten nights of six hours of sleep can double the risk of mental illness reinforces the significance of prioritizing sufficient, uninterrupted sleep.

Physical Activity

The last chapter discussed in detail the importance of exercising, mentioning it being a component of maintaining mental health. Exercise facilitates better oxygenation of the brain, positively influencing the function of the prefrontal cortex, and contributing to overall mental well-being.

Stress Management

If one follows a healthy and balanced diet, prioritizes sleep, and exercises regularly, then it has an advantage, and stress becomes easier to manage as everything is interconnected. Steering clear of unhealthy coping mechanisms, including excessive caffeine, alcohol, and tobacco use, while incorporating stress-reducing activities like mindfulness and exercise, forms a holistic strategy for stress management.

On top of those four areas, there are other important factors to take into consideration, like exposure to sunlight, which benefits our mood among other things. Having social connections and engaging in any social activity, creating a relationship with other humans, is also beneficial to our brain and overall well-being, as we are social by nature and could not live completely alone. If we could, we'd have an unhappy and unfulfilled life. Lastly, practices like yoga, meditation, and deep breathing are suggested for relaxation and stress reduction, emphasizing the holistic nature of well-being.

The importance of God

Barbara O`Neill is known to incorporate religious beliefs in some of her lectures. She often talks about the importance of God when talking about mental health. Emphasizing trust in God is highlighted as a source of peace and hope. She encourages relying on God's wisdom and guidance, especially in challenging situations that everyone encounters during life.

She believes that having faith in God during challenging times is a key aspect for our mental health. Sadly, in our lives, everyone happens to experience negativity, including grief, anxiety, discontent, remorse, guilt, and distrust. These feelings are normal, however, if they stay with us for long they can lead to physical changes in the brain, affecting not only our mental health but also our physical health. Another key aspect that Barbara mentions often is the physiological benefits of forgiveness. She explains that forgiveness cleanses the brain and frees individuals from the negative impact of past experiences. Some people struggle with forgiveness and tend to be tense and anxious or have other negative feelings that in the long term are very harmful to our mental health and overall well-being.

The good news is that regardless of your actual situation, you can change and improve. The brain is not hardwired; it is changeable through a process called neuroplasticity. This means that anyone can adapt and change. So, even if you struggle with certain positive beliefs or good habits, through consistent practice and effort all these things suggested by Barbara will become natural.

The importance of meditation and breathing

Barbara O'Neill emphasizes that the brain, akin to any other muscle, requires training, a practice often neglected by the majority of people. While not delving into precise details, she advocates various methods for brain training, including meditation, breathing, and prayer, highlighting the benefits of these practices.

In her teachings, Barbara underscores the calming effect of meditation on the mind, enhancing awareness. She refers to research that indicates consistent meditation as conducive to forming positive habits, alleviating stress and overthinking, preventing and helping dealing with anxiety, and fostering a greater sense of presence. Meditation also helps to find out more about yourself. Meditation, as explained by Barbara, is an excellent daily mental training. It has many benefits and it is suggested to improve mental clarity, emotional balance, and spiritual connection, promoting relaxation, reducing stress, and enhancing overall health. The incorporation of meditation into daily life aligns perfectly with Barbara O'Neill's holistic approach to health and wellness.

Regarding breathing, Barbara notes that many individuals may not engage in proper breathing techniques. She stresses the importance of breathing through the nose, elucidating that mouth breathing can be detrimental to overall well-being as it involves inhaling unpurified air, potentially laden with germs. Nose breathing is advocated for its role in purifying, humidifying, balancing blood gases, and pressurizing air, contributing to optimal oxygen intake. Barbara's viewpoint on breathing aligns with scientific understanding. Practicing deep breathing is very useful for calmness and to let go of stress and anxiety.

Barbara's religious beliefs are robust, and she emphasizes the advantages of prayer. Prayer can take various forms, with no specific wrong way to pray. She frequently highlights the potency of expressing gratitude and thankfulness in our prayers, asserting that it profoundly influences our emotions, especially when practiced consistently. Barbara firmly believes in the correlation between our physical well-being and spiritual development, praying contributes to creating a healthy and resilient mind.

Depression

Depression is a serious and complex topic experienced by many individuals daily. Barbara emphasizes that adopting a healthy lifestyle is crucial in preventing and fighting depression. She stresses the importance of a well-balanced diet, advocating for the inclusion of various foods such as plant-based options, proteins, grains, legumes, nuts, seeds, and healthy fats. Plant-based foods are praised for their nutritional richness, contributing to an improved sense of well-being, while proteins play a crucial role in supporting mood-regulating neurotransmitters, as explored in-depth earlier. Understanding this chapter is essential as it has far-reaching consequences in many other aspects.

Physical exercise is also highly beneficial. As discussed earlier, it comes in various forms and, among the numerous benefits mentioned before, strengthens mental resilience. This, in turn, encourages individuals to make mindful food choices that support both their physical and mental well-being.

As mentioned earlier, sunshine exposure is incredibly important for our well-being and mood. Therefore, it is particularly suggested for people who feel depressed. Sunlight helps the pineal gland release serotonin, which, as stated earlier, is a neurotransmitter linked with mood regulation. If you want a better mood, listen to Barbara and get some sunshine on your skin.

Barbara O'Neill provides a thorough exploration of various contributors to depression, examining substances and environmental factors that can significantly influence mental health, the main ones are :

- **Alcohol** : O'Neill categorizes alcohol as toxic for any human being, emphasizing its potential harm to the brain.

- **Tobacco** : Tobacco is not only harmful to our lungs, but breathing suboptimal air also poses challenges to our brain. In fact, it impacts the cognitive and emotional aspects of our health.

- **Drugs** : It is common knowledge that both legal and illegal mind-altering drugs are categorized as contributors to depression, and Barbara agrees with that.

- **Lack of sun exposure** : As explained earlier, sunshine is great for optimal mood and well-being, and being in nature is always beneficial for our health, in line with our human nature. Going against this law of nature always has a negative effect.

- **MSG (Monosodium Glutamate)** : The possible harmful effect of MSG on our nerves shows how stuff added to food can affect our nervous system, playing a role in how what we eat relates to our mental health.

- **Mold** : It has been mentioned earlier of various negative effects of mold and reasons why to avoid it. Living or spending time in a surrounding where mold is implies our health.

- **Electromagnetic Fields** : Considering excessive electromagnetic field exposure as a contributor introduces a less tangible but equally impactful element. This prompts contemplation of unnoticed environmental factors that may play a role in mental health challenges. No wonder that since there is more technology around and some people are immersed in it, there are more and more people having mental health problems.

Barbara O'Neill encourages deeper reflection on individuals' daily choices. Her approach to depression is holistic, emphasizing that there is no single cure or shortcut. It involves a combination of actions, including diet, sleep, exercise, and other aspects mentioned in the book so far.

Three shockers that stimulate the brain are :

1. **Breakfast like a king, lunch like a queen, and an 18-hour fast :** This method creates a shock to the body when it doesn't receive food. The fast, as explained by Barbara, functions as a shock for the mind, which is great.

2. **Hot shower, finish with a bit of cold water :** This contrasting temperature shower stimulates the body and provides a shock effect. This is something that has been mentioned in one of her interviews. Barbara explains that it is not necessary to keep the cold water for long; it is absolutely subjective to the timing. However, it is suggested to end with cold water, even for a little bit, to have that "shock feeling" that stimulates not only our body but our brain too.

3. **HIIT (High-Intensity Interval Training) :** Engaging in HIIT exercises provides a shock to the body, promoting increased heart rate and intense physical activity. It has been explained earlier the incredible benefits of HIIT.

Natural Remedies

In this chapter, we will explore several natural remedies for specific problems. However, it is important to understand that the key fundamentals of health that we have discussed so far are the most important things to prioritize. They are a necessary requirement for better health and form the basis for the most effective natural remedies for any issue.

The popularity of Barbara's teachings worldwide can be attributed mainly to natural remedies, which serve as the primary reason why she is widely listened to.

Before uncovering Barbara's teachings, we must take a step back and introduce a very fascinating concept that Barbaar mentions, which is "What causes certain diseases?" and what is the role of DNA.

The importance of DNA

Barbara introduces two main ideas as to what causes certain diseases to answer this question: the gene theory and the germ theory. In short, the germ theory suggests that external factors like germs are responsible for making people sick, taking away individual accountability. While, the gene theory attributes health problems to one's genes, further reducing personal responsibility.

So, your genes and DNA play a part in determining the diseases you might encounter in your life. While explaining the specific and complicated double-banded helix DNA structure she connects this structure to Hippocrates' saying: "Let food be thy medicine and medicine be thy food," emphasizing how the components of DNA align with the nutrients we get from our diet. Once again, emphasizing the importance of what we eat. This is not meant to be a biology or scientific book, so we will not delve deeper into the structure of DNA. However, it is important to know that DNA is incredibly fascinating and complex and O¬Neill explains that if its information were written out, it would fill thousands of books with thousands of pages each and around three thousand letters every page.

The human body can be seen as a collection of cells with various functions, including skin cells, tissue cells, and bone cells. Barbara explains that DNA serves as the genetic code defining individuality. The DNA comprises 23 chromosomes from both the mother and the father. Stressing the constant regeneration of cells, she mentions that within six months, a person virtually has a new body. As also explained in the introduction of the book, due to the varied rates at which cells are remade, achieving a completely new body might take longer, roughly two years according to Barbara.

Why do we use antibiotics and painkillers?

Barbara brings a viewpoint to the table. She introduces us to Antoine Béchamp, a figure in history who often gets overshadowed by Louis Pasteur. While Pasteur gained fame for his studies on the germ theory and the use of medications to combat germs Béchamp proposed a perspective. Béchamp emphasized the significance of lifestyle and nutrition in maintaining health. He highlighted how our internal environment plays a role in determining our well being. Despite Béchamps insights Pasteur's germ theory gained popularity, which eventually led to the widespread usage of antibiotics and antimicrobial drugs, in modern medicine.

Pain

Pain is debilitating, anyone who has ever experienced pain knows that it is a very uncomfortable experience and we would prefer avoiding it. The mainstream makes us use painkillers when we have some pain. Barbara's holistic and natural view is against the use of medicine such as painkillers when we have pain. Opting for more natural options.

Barbara emphasises the need to investigate the cause of pain, referencing Newton's third law of motion, which states that "for every action, there is an equal and opposite reaction", and the biblical principle that "the curse causeless shall not come", which suggests that negative consequence doesn't happen without a reason or cause.

Focusing on the root cause is the key to avoiding dependence on painkillers and breaking free from a cycle of pain. She emphasizes the importance of understanding a person's history, injuries, and lifestyle factors in effectively addressing pain, recognizing that everyone is unique and responds differently.

Hot and Cold treatment

Barbara introduces the concept of hot and cold treatments as one of the easiest and most common natural remedies. Explaining their effectiveness in stimulating blood flow, reducing inflammation, and promoting healing. She often combines using the hot and cold treatment with using comfrey poultices, highlighting its growth-stimulating and anti-inflammatory properties. For instance, she narrates that a powerful way to fix plantar fasciitis is using hot and cold treatments along with comfrey cream for relief.

The role of Ice

Barbara emphasizes the significant role of ice in reducing inflammation and aiding the recovery process. Applying ice can be beneficial in different situations as it serves to cool down the inflammation and bring relief. When discussing her foot injury during a skydiving incident, she highlights the use of ice to alleviate swelling and manage pain effectively. By using ice, Barbara effectively reduces the swelling around her injured foot.

Barbara's experience with ice shows its role as a natural and accessible method for anyone to manage inflammation and promote healing in the context of pain relief.

However, she emphasizes the importance of listening to the body's response and adjusting the ice application accordingly as we all differ and some people can then have different reactions to the application of ice in injuries.

So far, we have seen many of Barbara O'Neill's teachings. The knowledge you acquire is precious, and if you consistently apply her suggestions, you will see your life completely transformed. Her teachings are very holistic and natural. It has been mentioned so far of some food, element, and lifestyle advice that is incredibly helpful for certain conditions. Now, I'd like to simplify it for you, by starting with the issues that someone can face and the actions to take according to the studies conducted on the subject. This chapter is a true gold as it can literally drastically change your life and your perspective on some health issues.

Natural Remedies for Flu and Bronchitis

The flu is one of the most common illnesses that circulates every year. However, many people are unsure about how to combat it and often resort to taking pills. Barbara has a solution to your problems – she has created a natural remedy known as the "Flu Bomb." This remedy is not only effective against the flu but can also be used for other issues like bronchitis, asthma, and sinus problems.

Here are the ingredients needed to make the Flu Bomb:

- Crushed garlic (the amount depends on your comfort level)
- Finely grated ginger (about one-quarter of a tablespoon)
- Eucalyptus oil (or Tea Tree oil if you don't have the former)
- One drop of cayenne pepper (from one-quarter to half a teaspoon, depending on your tolerance)

This natural remedy offers an alternative to traditional medications, providing a holistic approach to tackling various respiratory issues. Remember to adjust the quantities of ingredients based on your personal preferences and tolerances.

Barbara points out that often people who chronically feel sick or tired in the morning are due to a magnesium deficiency. She, therefore, suggests consuming food rich in magnesium like green leafy vegetables, avocado, nuts, legumes and many others mentioned in the last chapters already.

Hydrotherapy

Hydrotherapy is also a great option for enhancing overall health. Therefore, it is suggested that it can take various forms:

- Warm baths or showers help relax muscles, alleviate stress, and can assist in lowering temperature.
- Cold baths and showers are used to reduce inflammation.
- Contrast hydrotherapy involves alternating between hot and cold water to stimulate circulation, enhancing overall health.

Natural Remedies for Managing Chronic Pain

Millions of people worldwide suffer from chronic pain. According to Barbara, this is primarily attributed to lifestyle choices, as observed thus far, and the fact that singular problems are often treated rather than addressing the root cause, failing to consider the body in a holistic manner. In reality, people frequently resort to painkillers, as explained earlier, which might alleviate the problem momentarily but does not ensure a lasting solution.

Barbara presents various options for different problems, the following are the most frequently mentioned solutions:

Ginger

Ginger is highly recommended for joint inflammation, as it is a powerful anti-inflammatory herb. Its benefits extend beyond consumption, as applying it externally to areas of inflammation can be highly effective. O'Neill emphasizes the remarkable benefits of applying a ginger poultice to areas with inflammation. This practice is encouraged because ginger pulls the inflammation from the joint to the skin, causing the skin to become warm. Here's how to create a ginger poultice :

1. Take a plate.
2. Place a small plastic backing on it to prevent it from wetting your skin.
3. Lay a cloth over the plate.
4. Grate ginger onto the cloth.

This method is particularly beneficial for joint inflammation, gout, or arthritis, providing a natural and potentially soothing remedy.

Potato

Potatoes are not just considered as a food by Barbara; she acknowledges their various beneficial uses. Potatoes are highly optimal for tissue inflammation. Barbara recommends them for reducing swelling and addressing inflammation of the skin, as well as for cooling and soothing inflamed eyes, such as in cases of conjunctivitis.

Potatoes can also be effectively used fo r:

- Ankle sprains
- Gout
- Arthritis

The richness of potassium and phosphorus in potatoes makes them alkaline in nature, contributing to their anti-inflammatory effects. They play a role in reducing inflammation and promoting overall healing. Barbara suggests combining potatoes with hot and cold treatments to maximize inflammation reduction.

Here's how to make a potato poultice and use it :

1. The process of making a potato poultice can be mess-free by using plastic wrap and a disposable cleaning cloth.
2. Grate the potato directly onto the cloth, ensuring even coverage.
3. Fold the cloth over the grated potato to create a poultice package.
4. Apply the poultice to the affected area, securing it with bandages if necessary.
5. For added relief, consider incorporating hot and cold hydrotherapy before or after applying the poultice.

It's important to note that poultices may need to be applied regularly until the desired results are achieved. In conclusion, potatoes are versatile and can be effectively used for a range of tissue inflammations, providing a natural and non-invasive approach to healing.

Cayenne pepper

Cayenne pepper has several benefits that have also been mentioned earlier. Barbara explains that it can be extremely beneficial for fighting and finding relief from back pain. In fact, using cayenne while cooking and incorporating it into your diet serves as a natural painkiller.

Onion

As explained before, onions have several benefits, among which is the chance to alleviate chest cold or head cold symptoms. In fact, by placing an onion in a plastic bag on your feet and then putting socks on, it helps in curing chest and head colds.

This happens because onions have antimicrobial properties, and when applied to the feet, they are believed to be absorbed into the bloodstream, promoting the body's natural healing processes. Barbara's theory is fascinating, and some people report benefiting from this practice. However, it is important to note that individual experiences may vary. There is no scientific evidence supporting the effectiveness of this method; however, according to O'Neill's experience and studies, it can be an effective way to alleviate certain illnesses.

Hydrotherapy

As explained earlier, Hydrotherapy has several health benefits and it is also very used for fighting chronic pain. The contrast between hot and cold is optimal for chronic pain relief and promotes faster healing.

Natural Remedies for Skin Health Problems

Barbara believes that every skin disease has an allergy component. So, whenever there is a skin problem, such as eczema, psoriasis, rosacea, it is suggested to eliminate the five allergens:

- Diary
- Wheat
- Oat
- Peanuts
- Refined sugar

Once we take actions to fix these problems, it is a process of trials and errors until we find a solution. Therefore, it is necessary to be patient with results, as it takes at least 2 months to see results coming from this change of diet. Barbara stresses the importance of understanding that many people want a "quick fix," and that is not always the case for lasting and effective changes.

In addition to the five allergens, there is another factor that can affect skin problems, that is "Hormonal Imbalance".

59

Hormonal Imbalance

Barbara O'Neill suggests that hormonal imbalance, specifically having high estrogen and low progesterone levels, can contribute to skin problems. As hormones play a crucial role in regulating various bodily functions, including skin health. Barbar explains that whenever there is an imbalance, it can lead to issues such as acne, eczema, or other skin conditions.

High estrogen levels relative to progesterone are a common example of hormone imbalance, this can be impacted by:

- Stress
- Diet
- Lifestyle
- Sleep
- Sunlight

Mold

Another factor that can cause skin problems is mold exposure in the house or in the place where it is spent during the day. The problem of mold are several and have been discussed deeply in the book.
As you can see, the main natural remedies for bone and skin health are diet and lifestyle choices, which are the focus of Barbara's teachings.

Castor oil

Arguably, the worst skin issue is skin cancer and skin moles. For this problem, Barbara discovered a powerful way to fight it. In fact, castor oil represents an incredibly powerful remedy. Various examples brought by Barbara show that putting a dab of castor oil every day can be very effective for skin cancer.

Natural Remedies for Bone Health

Healthy bones are strong bones, and to have strong bones, it is necessary to include in our diet a substantial dose of calcium. Barbara does not approve of calcium supplements, as those can be considered harmful for the mineral balance. She, in fact, in line with her holistic view, suggests consuming not only calcium but also underscores the importance of the minerals that compose the bones such as magnesium and zinc.

She emphasizes the importance of obtaining these minerals from natural sources. Dark green leafy vegetables, such as kale and spinach. She explains that even in the case of injuries if we have in our body the right minerals the healing process can happen naturally and easily without the need for pills.

On top of that, she has a fascinating and effective natural remedy, a special cream, the Yan cream.

Yan Cream

Osteoporosis is a medical condition characterized by the weakening of the bones. According to Barbara, it is caused by an imbalance, often caused by low progesterone, which is the hormone that boosts bone-building cells. By using the Yam Cream, this problem can be fixed. Yam cream is often mentioned by Barbara as a natural remedy because it contains diosgenin. Applying diosgenin on our skin makes it get in touch with fat cells on the skin, stimulating the pathway that our body uses to make progesterone. So, the Yam cream works with the body to stimulate the increase of progesterone, boosting bone-building cells and therefore bone health.

This cream is suggested to be applied morning and night. For women, twice a day for three weeks when not menstruating, as during that time of the month progesterone levels are naturally high. How much should be applied? One finger dip up until the nail bed, just a little dip, and apply: inside of arms, chest, inside of thighs, and abdomen. Apply it only in one area and then the following time that you apply the cream apply it in a different area.

Natural Remedies for Gut and Liver Health

By now you should know what are the main actions to take to have a healthy body. Things like a high-fiber diet, staying hydrated, and engaging in regular exercise promote gut and liver health as explained numerous times by Barbara. A crucial lesson Barbara O'Neill imparts is the significant connection between gut health, inflammation, and the alkaline-acid balance. For a deeper understanding of this aspect, I encourage you to explore that specific chapter.

Gut health is an extremely important topic to Barbara, and she shows that every time during her health retreats where she talks about gut healing. Barbara devised a holistic strategy incorporating Slippery Elm and probiotics administered four times daily. This plan is coupled with the elimination of wheat, dairy, refined sugar, and alcohol from the patient's diet. Encouraging results become evident within a week, showcasing a reduction in bowel movements from six to three times a day, accompanied by the cessation of bleeding and cramping.

Slippery Elm

Slippery elm is an herb often mentioned by Barbara. It is a versatile substance that can be used both internally and externally. When mixed with water, it forms a jelly-like consistency similar to mucus. Ingested, it coats and soothes the entire gastrointestinal tract, providing relief for issues from sore throat to ulcerated stomach. With a gentle stimulant effect, it promotes rapid healing in the digestive system. Overall, slippery elm proves to be a beneficial remedy for various gastrointestinal conditions, offering both soothing and healing properties.

Another important concept for optimal gut health is understanding enzymes. They are crucial for a healthy gut as they help break down food, facilitating the absorption of essential nutrients. Enzymes play a key role in digestion and overall gut well-being. Enzyme-rich foods include lemon, cayenne pepper, pineapple, papaya, dandelions, gentian, and St. Mary's thistle.

Barbara's advice is to eliminate problematic foods, offering a potential remedy for various gut issues. Practical tips for maintaining colon and gut health include herbal remedies, hydrotherapy, and adopting proper toilet posture.

Herbal Remedies

Barbara O'Neill frequently discusses the incorporation of specific herbs into her plant-based diet to enhance digestive health. Her dietary choices align with utilizing the diverse properties that herbs offer, contributing to various aspects of gastrointestinal well-being, including aiding digestion, reducing inflammation, and promoting overall gut health.

Among the herbs highlighted by O'Neill for their digestive benefits are :

- Ginger
- Peppermint
- Aloe Vera

These herbs can be incorporated into one's diet in different forms, such as teas, tinctures, or supplements, providing flexibility for individuals to choose the method that suits them best.

O'Neill underscores the importance of selecting herbal remedies based on individual needs and conditions. Different people may experience varying degrees of benefit from specific herbs, emphasizing the personalized nature of herbal supplementation. Seeking guidance from healthcare professionals or herbalists can help tailor herbal choices to align with individual health goals and requirements.

Hydrotherapy

Barbara O'Neill sees hydrotherapy as a valuable tool for promoting gut health. Alternating hot and cold showers enhance circulation and support the digestive system's function. If we apply Hot and cold compresses on the abdominal area this has a positive impact on digestion and detoxification.

Proper Toilet Posture

Barbara emphasizes the importance of adopting a natural squatting position during bowel movements. This posture is considered more aligned with the body's natural mechanics, opposite to sitting.

While the scientific evidence supporting the benefits of squatting over sitting is limited, some individuals report improved bowel movements and reduced straining when adopting this posture.

It's essential for individuals to understand how their body reacts to herbal remedies, hydrotherapy, and changes in toilet posture. Consulting with a qualified practitioner is recommended for personalized advice, taking into account individual health conditions and specific needs.

Barbara O'Neill discusses the crucial role of the liver in maintaining overall health, emphasizing its importance in preventing diseases like cancer and promoting a healthy body. She highlights the liver's resilience due to its ability to regenerate. O'Neill also addresses the issue of high carbohydrate consumption in modern diets, particularly in America, and its impact on blood glucose levels and insulin release. She suggests that reducing carbohydrate intake can lead to positive health outcomes, emphasizing the liver's role in regulating carbohydrates in the body.

Barbara discusses the Atkins diet, which emphasizes low carbohydrates and high protein and fat. She promotes a diet low in carbohydrates for various health reasons, particularly for a healthier liver. However, she advises against eliminating carbohydrates completely, explaining that the issue with carbohydrates lies in their refinement and overconsumption. The speaker suggests adjusting the ratio of carbohydrates in meals based on factors such as age, size, and physical activity level.

Lemon

As explained earlier, lemon is one of the best tonics for the liver, and it also alkalizes the tissues, making it great in the morning with warm water.

Having lemon with a bit of boiling water before a meal is a great digestive aid. While lemon is acidic, it serves as an excellent digestive aid and promotes weight loss.

Another thing that can be done is taking 1/4 teaspoons of cayenne pepper in a glass with a small amount of water before the meal. It might feel like a burn, but it never burns. It might tingle, but it also wakes up the gastric glands, increasing the body's ability to digest.

Natural Remedies For Cancer

As usual, Barbara O'Neill provides a holistic perspective on preventing and battling cancer through natural remedies, stressing the significance of lifestyle. In terms of food, an aspect extremely important for the prevention of cancer is eliminating processed options. She suggests herbal supplements like essiac tea, Graviola, and turmeric. The importance of creating an alkaline body environment is a concept that's been dealt with earlier and is extremely important again in this situation.

Natural remedies, such as Anna's Wild Yam Cream, are suggested for hormone balance, particularly for reproductive system cancers.

Barbara suggests that cancer thrives in acidic, oxygen-deprived environments and thrives on sugar. To counteract this, she proposes alkalizing the tissues, promoting oxygenation in the body, and advocating for the elimination or significant reduction of glucose.

Castor Oil

Castor oil is by far one of the most mentioned elements by O`Neill when talking about diseases. She talks about castor oil often due to its pretty awesome benefits which often leave people mind-blown. Castor oil applied on the skin can go deep into your body and help with the following things :

- Lumps
- Bumps
- Fibroids
- Cysts
- Bone spurs
- Skin cancer

Considering the thickness of the oil it can be used as a pack, especially on your belly for problems with your uterus, ovaries, or colon.

Gallstones, kidney stones, and bone spurs can be annoying and painful issues. By putting the oil on the areas that need help, it can go deep and help them get better. Castor oil is part of a healthy lifestyle that can help with different health problems, even ones related to your brain or bones. Therefore, it is perfect for those who want to follow a natural and holistic lifestyle.

Castor oil can be used in two main ways. The first involves applying a dab of castor oil daily, which can be very effective for skin cancer. The second method is using it as a pack for a few hours each day over several days or weeks, and it can yield positive results. The same pack can be reused multiple times. Castor oil is overall considered an oil that can be bought at an affordable price. Reusing the pack a few times is mentioned by Barbar as an option considering that it would still benefit you. Whether you're dealing with problems inside your body or on your skin, castor oil is great because it goes deep and can help.

Castor oil must not be ingested. Barbara emphasizes this point several times, stating that castor oil should not be consumed.
The benefits of castor oil are incredible, by using castor oil people experience breast lumps get smaller, tumors go away for example.

Herbs and Cancer

Earlier in the chapter "Diet" it has been stated the Hydrangea Analogy, explaining the role of a good pH in cancer.That shows us that in order to avoid cancer it is necessary to avoid diets rich in processed foods, sugars, and unhealthy fats contribute to acidity, creating a potential breeding ground for various diseases, including cancer. Conversely, adopting an alkaline-promoting diet that emphasizes fruits, vegetables, and whole foods creates an environment less favorable for cancer growth.

Barbara recommends the herb Red Clover as a means to maintain a balanced internal pH. Red Clover is rich in phytochemicals, and incorporating this herb into our diet can be beneficial for preventing and managing cancer.

In conclusion, holistic nutrition stresses the role of antioxidants in preventing cancer. Colorful fruits and veggies, rich in antioxidants, protect against cellular damage. Mindful eating, a holistic practice, enhances digestion and well-being, forming a crucial part of cancer prevention.

Natural Remedies for Stomach Health

In the case of stomach tumors, Barbara suggests using Aloe vera and myrrh for healing when antibiotics are not available.

To avoid stomach problems, it is recommended to refrain from overeating, experiencing fear or anger, and consuming excessive fluids with meals, as these factors can hinder digestion. Moreover, giving the stomach a rest between meals is crucial for effective digestion and nutrient absorption. Therefore, it is important not to overeat, and Barbara strongly advocates for occasional fasting.

Another key aspect for stomach health is the consumption of water. Barbara often emphasizes the importance of water, specifically mentioning its benefits for the stomach. In fact, she shares a story about a man who was suffering from stomach pain, and the main cause was dehydration. After starting to drink more water on a daily basis (Barbara suggests roughly 2 liters), the stomach pain disappeared.

Stomach health is crucial for breaking down proteins and extracting nutrients for the body's nourishment. As you probably already understand, Barbara is a strong believer that everything is interconnected; neglecting one aspect may have implications elsewhere.

Natural Remedies For Heart Disease

The heart is arguably the most important muscle in our body; everything starts and ends there. In addition to maintaining a healthy lifestyle, it is crucial to shift away from processed foods and prioritize whole, plant-based nutrition, emphasizing fruits, vegetables, whole grains, and legumes. Barbara often emphasizes the importance of absolutely avoiding stress, as it is considered one of the main causes of heart diseases.

Certain foods serve as excellent remedies and prevention for heart diseases.

Cayenne pepper

The healing properties of cayenne pepper have already been mentioned. Beyond its association with spiciness, it emerges as a powerful circulatory stimulant, demonstrating healing capabilities for stomach ulcers and significantly promoting blood circulation, thereby preventing heart disease.

Hawthorn Berry Tea

Hawthorn berry tea is considered a beneficial herbal supplement, and regular consumption is optimal for regulating blood pressure and promoting heart health. It is by far the most mentioned herb when talking about the heart. Its benefits extend to managing blood circulation and promoting overall health. Barbara provides several examples of people who have had strokes and have gradually improved by consuming this herb.

Garlic

Garlic has cardiovascular benefits and it is linked to reducing blood pressure and cholesterol levels.

Motherwort

Motherwort helps ease nervous tension and calms the cardiovascular system. This is a typical example of an herb mentioned by Barbara that aligns with holistic principles, recognizing the interconnectedness of well-being.

Dandelion

Dandelion, often dismissed as a common weed, boasts diuretic properties that contribute to cardiovascular health by promoting a healthy fluid balance.

Natural Remedies for Headaches

Firstly, Barbara suggests the most common and easiest option to prevent and cure headaches, which is drinking water. She attributes headaches to a lack of water and addresses the problem accordingly.

She also provides other remedies to alleviate different types of aches, such as earaches. In fact, she narrates a story where her daughter used an onion poultice, leveraging the numerous benefits of onions.

The preparation of the onion in this case is again easy: steaming an onion and applying it to the ear provided quick relief. This success led Barbara to explore natural remedies further.

Barbara encourages listening to the body's signals and understanding the signs of improvement. In summary, the application of a warm, cooked onion poultice on the ear is a natural remedy for earaches, offering relief and aiding the body's healing process.

In addition to drinking more water and harnessing the power of onions to alleviate headaches, Barbara frequently underscores the significance of sleep in relation to this topic. She emphasizes the importance of avoiding the use of technological devices before bedtime. By refraining from this habit, among its many benefits, one can reduce the likelihood of waking up with a headache.

Natural Remedies For Diabetes

When discussing diabetes, it is necessary to mention glucose. Managing glucose levels is key, and Barbara starts by providing a few common tips that can be summarized as follows :

- Avoid refined sugar and wheat.
- Do not exceed carbohydrates like pasta, pizza, bread, or cereals.

Like other health issues, it is crucial to follow an alkaline diet, exercise consistently, stay hydrated, prioritize sleep, and maintain healthy routines to give yourself a better chance for healing. Specifically, understanding how blood sugar affects diabetes is essential, emphasizing the impact of food choices and diet on blood sugar levels.

Therefore, Barbara's primary advice for naturally addressing diabetes is to initially eliminate unhealthy sugars, such as palm sugar, maple syrup, and honey, until the pancreas begins to recover. It's important to note that Barbara is not against the consumption of organic honey; in fact, quite the opposite. However, for individuals with diabetes, she suggests temporarily removing it from the diet.

Eliminating refined sugar from the diet is crucial in preventing and combating diabetes. Barbara's enlightening studies emphasize that to avoid spikes in glucose, it is necessary to follow a specific order in meals :
1. Start with vegetables.
2. Follow with proteins and fats.
3. Conclude with starches and sugar.

Barbara believes that cow's milk is one of the reasons why people develop diabetes. She advises against drinking it, as she contends that many individuals struggle to digest milk, leading to proteins entering the bloodstream. According to Barbara, this can trigger an immune system response, potentially affecting the pancreas and becoming a contributing factor to diabetes. Barbara's reasoning is clear and logical; therefore, she suggests avoiding the consumption of cow's milk.

Legumes, on the contrary, are very advisable for diabetic people because they have a low glycemic index. Legumes like chickpeas, lentils, or black-eyed beans contribute to better blood sugar control, which makes them fundamental in one's diet.

In one of her lectures, Barbara shared a case study involving a young man named Dan, diagnosed with type 1 diabetes at 15 due to antibiotics. The program showcased positive results. Dan's improvement was notable after he stopped consuming wheat, caffeine, and refined sugar, as caffeine can trigger an insulin response. Following these dietary changes, he experienced significant improvements in his overall health and the recovery of his pancreas.

In addition to the dietary recommendations outlined so far, it is crucial to follow the guidelines provided in the book, such as exercising and staying hydrated. Barbara emphasizes the importance of patience and having faith when addressing health issues.

Natural Remedies for Weight Loss

Weight loss is one of the most common topics in everyday life, regardless of age and gender. Many people wake up hoping to lose weight and may even try. However, due to mainstream ideas, often conflicting with each other, some people struggle a lot with this or put in an incredible amount of effort for small results, believing that it is the only way. Barbara emphasizes the importance of several things that have already been mentioned in the book so far, but for a better understanding, they will be mentioned again:

Diet

First of all, avoiding fats, as the mainstream often suggests, is not advisable. While some processed products containing "bad" fats should be avoided, other healthy fats like olive oil, coconut oil, and avocado are highly recommended in the diet. Coconut oil is claimed to aid weight loss.

Moreover, it is necessary to maintain a high-fiber diet by consuming vegetables. Including grains with a low glycemic index (GI) such as quinoa, millet, spelt, and buckwheat is extremely beneficial for weight loss. She also advises consuming legumes, a good source of protein, which is extremely beneficial for weight loss.

Barbara follows a plant-based diet, which she claims is optimal for weight loss. However, she recognizes that many people fail to understand that a plant-based diet has benefits only if followed properly, ensuring not only the inclusion of minerals and vitamins but also a sufficient amount of proteins and fats.

Barbara also advises us to double-check "Gluten-free" products, as they often tend to hide traces of refined sugar, inviting readers to make mindful decisions.

Another key tip is to drink lemon juice before eating.

Exercising

Obviously, in order to lose weight, she understands and emphasizes the importance of burning calories and engaging in exercises. As explained in the section on exercises, she suggests HIIT and rebounding.

Natural Remedies for Hormonal Imbalance

Barbara O'Neil focuses many of her lectures on hormonal imbalances, explaining their symptoms, causes, and potential solutions. She delves into the key hormones of the monthly cycle: estrogen and progesterone.

Barbara introduces the concept of "The pill," containing synthetic estrogen and progesterone. Over time, it has been linked to issues such as estrogen dominance and progesterone deficiency, leading to health problems like polyps, fibroids, cysts, and hormonal cancers. As a result, she advises against taking the pill, considering it harmful to the body.

The increasing use of plastics over the years has impacted hormonal balance as they contain substances like fennel that can mimic estrogen, contributing to elevated estrogen levels. Barbara recommends avoiding plastic containers, especially for hot soups, and being cautious with synthetic fabrics such as those used in bras.

Adopting a plant-based diet is promoted by Barbara as a means to encourage hormonal balance. In addition to dietary changes, she emphasizes the importance of lifestyle modifications and the elimination of certain substances to address hormonal imbalances.

Yam Cream

Anna's Wild Yam Cream is suggested to enhance progesterone levels. Emphasizing the body's innate ability to heal under the right conditions, she discourages unnecessary medical interventions, such as the removal of body parts. The speaker advises consulting with qualified healthcare professionals for personalized advice.

Natural Remedies for Cleaning

Maintaining a clean environment where we live or spend most of our time is beneficial to us in many ways. In fact, a chemical-free home enables us to breathe better, promoting a healthier house and body. Alternatives to those products are :

- **White Vinegar :** White Vinegar is a great natural disinfectant that helps remove stains and odors.

- **Olive Oil :** Olive Oil mixed with lemon juice, can be used to polish furniture, offering a great alternative to commonly used chemicals that perform the same job but may potentially harm our health.

- **Baking Soda :** Baking Soda is a mild abrasive that effectively cleans surfaces and helps eliminate odors.

Natural Remedies for Teeth

Barbara discusses the unique ability of teeth to heal themselves and emphasizes the importance of providing the right conditions for this healing process. She emphasizes the importance of making mindful choices regarding lifestyle, including fresh air, sunlight, enough sleep, exercise, and a nutritious diet.

Barbara highlights the role of food caught between teeth, which can lead to decay and damage. She recommends a couple of things to support dental health :

- Thorough rinsing
- Flossing after meals
- Oil pulling using Coconut Oil.

Barbara also emphasizes the importance of crunchy foods, like apples and raw vegetables, to strengthen the teeth, jaws, and gums. Some people tend not to eat crunchy foods scared that their teeth will be ruined, Barbara claims the opposite.

Ultimately, Barbara explains that it is important to focus on dental hygiene to potentially reduce the need for expensive dental treatments.

Natural Remedies for Hair

As explained by Barbara genetics play a significant role in determining hair color. When getting older, the majority of people tend to get gray hair. Barbara claims that consuming green food, also in the form of juices, which are a big source of minerals, can significantly slow down the graying of the hair. She suggests :

- Chlorophyll
- Green barley powder
- Wheatgrass powder

She also suggests not to throw away the water you use to cook these foods. The used water is rich in minerals, as she says that water can contribute to avoiding hair loss. To nourish your hair, O`Neill suggests trying a monthly coconut oil rub. The best way to apply it is to leave it in for a day and then shampoo it out. This is considered a fantastic and natural scalp treatment.

Hair loss is promoted by shampoos with lauryl sulfate, therefore she suggests making mindful choices to avoid those.

In summary, nurture your hair from within with a mineral-rich diet, avoid harmful chemicals, and treat your hair kindly with natural remedies.

Natural Remedies to Strengthen Pelvic floor

Yoni Stones are useful for strengthening the pelvic floor, increasing blood flow, and reviving and strengthening the pelvic girdle internally.

Barbara's daughter, Emma, gave birth to twin girls 18 years ago. Despite being advised to have a Cesarean section due to the twins being six pounds each, Emma insisted on having her babies naturally. However, she faced a common postpartum issue where laughter or coughing would lead to a bit of urine leakage. Emma was concerned about this and discovered Yoni Stones.

After wearing the Yoni Stones for three months, Emma noticed a significant improvement. The stones work by strengthening the pelvic girdle internally as they are worn. The recommended process involves starting with the largest stone, wearing it for increasing durations over several weeks, and gradually progressing to smaller stones. She suggests starting with one hour a day for a week as a start and gradually progressing one more hour a day until reaching a maximum of 5 hours a day.

This process helps strengthen the pelvic girdle, allowing the wearer to regain control over urinary functions. The stones are not magical; they simply assist in the internal strengthening of the pelvic muscles.
On top of this, Yoni stones are also used by those women who experience pain during sex. Barbara explains stories of women that after consistently using Yoni stones started to stop feeling pain during sex.

Yoni stones suggested by Barbara have not yet had many scientific resources behind them so Barbara suggests seeing how your body reacts to them.

Recipes

Planning meals is vital to avoid overeating and making conscious, mindful decisions about what to eat, as emphasized in O'Neill's teachings, as we have covered so far.

She mentioned numerous times that she eats twice a day: she has breakfast, which is her "Fruit Meal," and lunch, which is her "Vegetables Meal." She rarely eats at night, and when she does, it is very light. Her meals are often accompanied by drinking lemon juice with a bit of boiling water before starting eating. This combination is said to boost digestion.

In this chapter, we will go through a few of the recipes suggested by Barbara in her meals.

Obviously, the following recipes are just a few suggestions. By reading the book so far, you should be able to know what kind of food to eat and create your recipes. These recipes are simply ideas and follow guidelines; Barbara's teachings do not intend to make people eat exactly what she eats. Adjust your diet according to your preferences.

Breakfast Recipes

Barbara advises to "have breakfast like a king," implying a substantial morning meal. As mentioned earlier, Barbara typically opts for fruit-based breakfasts. Chia seeds are a consistent part of her morning routine due to their optimal properties for a breakfast meal.

Avocado Toast with Fruit and Legume Delight

Ingredients :

- 2 or 3 pieces of your favorite fruits (e.g., berries, apple slices, or banana)
- Sourdough spelt toast
- Olive oil (for drizzling)
- 1 ripe avocado
- Your choice of legumes (red lentils, brown lentils, black-eyed beans, or scrambled organic tofu)
- Assorted nuts and seeds

Instructions :

1. Prepare the Avocado Toast : Toast the sourdough spelt bread to your liking, then slice the ripe avocado and arrange the slices on top of the toasted bread before drizzling olive oil over the avocado.

2. Create the Legume Delight : Choose your preferred legume (red lentils, brown lentils, black-eyed beans, or scrambled organic tofu), prepare it according to your preference (cooked, sautéed, or scrambled), and then mix in assorted nuts and seeds for added texture and flavor.

3. Assemble the Breakfast : Place the Avocado Toast on your plate, arrange the selected fruits around the toast, and serve the Legume Delight alongside.

Notes : Barbara mentioned that this breakfast is the most frequently chosen daily option.

Low-Sugar Smoothie

Ingredients :

- 1 cup of fluid (e.g., soy milk, almond milk, or coconut water)
- Berries, that add flavour and fiber to the meal
- Avocado for creaminess, minerals, and healthy fats
- Nuts and seeds for additional healthy fats and protein (Chia seeds or ground flax seeds)
- Protein powder for increased protein content (pea, hemp, or organic soy without sweeteners)

- Dessert spoon of coconut cream or coconut oil for added creaminess and flavor
- Dessert spoon of carob powder for complex carbohydrates and a bit of protein

Instructions :
Place all ingredients in a blender and blend it and adjust the thickness or sweetness by adding more or less fluid or organic sweeteners.

Notes : This smoothie suggested by Barbara as an optimal breakfast appears to be a well-rounded meal as it provides a mix of macronutrients, healthy fats, protein, and fiber.

Chia Seed Pudding

Ingredients:

- Chia seeds
- Nut milk (cashew milk used)
- Truvani vanilla protein powder
- Raspberries
- Lemon Juice (optional)

Instructions:

Whisk chia seeds with nut milk, blend in Truvani vanilla protein powder, add optional lemon juice, pour into a mason jar, and top with mashed raspberries.

Notes: Barbara mentions that these chia seed puddings are one of the most eaten breakfasts by the people who go to her retreats. Probably because of its tastiness and nutritional properties.

Berry and Grain Breakfast

Ingredients:

- Low GI fruits (e.g., blackberries, blueberries, cherries)
- Grains (e.g., oats or millet)
- Stewed Granny Smith apples (optional, for sweetness)
- Stevia (as a natural sweetener, to taste)
- Coconut milk or nut milk (almond, soy, or cashew)
- Ground flax seeds
- Nuts (e.g., almonds)

Instructions:

Prepare the grains (such, as oats or millet) following the instructions, on the package. Combine them with index fruits and cooked Granny Smith apples. If desired add a touch of stevia for sweetness. Pour coconut milk or nut milk over the mixture. Sprinkle ground flax. Top it off with some nuts.

Berry Protein Smoothie

Ingredients:

- 1 cup coconut water or almond/soy milk
- 1 dessert spoon of protein powder (brown rice or pea protein)
- 1 dessert spoon of coconut milk
- Berries (blackberries, blueberries, etc.)
- Chia seeds
- Ground flax seeds
- Green leaves (spinach or kale) (Optional)

Instructions:

To create a smoothie start by combining coconut water or milk with protein powder and coconut milk. Blend the mixture until it becomes smooth and creamy. Then incorporate berries, chia seeds, ground flax seeds and if you like some leaves. Blend everything together until you achieve your desired thickness. Finally pour the smoothie into a glass.

Sourdough Spelt Toast or Waffle

Ingredients:

- Sourdough spelt toast or waffle (made from soy or chickpea flour)
- Olive oil, coconut oil, or avocado (for spreading)
- Toppings: Savory lentils, scrambled tofu, sliced tomato, avocado, and a handful of nuts

Instructions:

You can start by toasting some sourdough spelt bread or making a waffle. Afterward, spread either olive oil or coconut oil on it. Even layer it with avocado. Next you can add your toppings such as lentils, scrambled tofu, sliced tomato and nuts.

Sunflower Sauce/Dressing

Ingredients:

- Sunflower seeds
- Water
- Lemon
- Garlic
- Salt

Instructions :

Blend sunflower seeds with water, lemon, garlic, and salt until smooth.

Notes : This breakfast option is suggested for someone who does not want to eat heavily and is looking for a very light breakfast. It is great for digestion as it is light and healthy and also has anti-inflammatory properties.

Keto Breakfast

Ingredients :

- Tomato
- Cucumber
- Avocado
- Olive oil
- Nuts
- Chocolate made with coconut oil, carob powder, and tahini (Optionally)

Notes : This breakfast is suggested by Barbara because it is high in fiber, fantastic for fast energy, and contains proteins, as well as many minerals and vitamins. Therefore, it is a great option for an energy-boosting diet.

Blueberry Jam

Ingredients:

- Wild blueberries
- Arrowroot (to thicken)
- Maple syrup or honey (optional)

Instructions:

Heat wild blueberries in a little water. Optionally, add maple syrup or honey for sweetness.

Notes: Barbara mentioned it as an option for those who enjoy a berry sauce. Blueberries are a great choice, offering antioxidant and anti-inflammatory properties, as well as being rich in fiber.

Homemade Granola Recipe

Ingredients:

- 6 cups regular rolled oats
- 3 cups quick oats
- 3/4 cup pecans
- 3/4 cup almonds
- 3/4 cup walnuts
- 1 1/2 cups dehydrated coconut
- 1 cup extra light olive oil (or liquefied coconut oil)
- 1 1/2 cups pineapple juice (or orange juice)
- 1 cup maple syrup
- 1 tablespoon pure vanilla
- Optional: Add raisins, dates, or dried pineapple after baking.

Instructions:

1. Prepare Dry Ingredients : Mix regular rolled oats, quick oats, pecans, almonds, walnuts, and dehydrated coconut in a bowl.

2. Prepare Wet Ingredients : In a separate bowl, combine olive oil (or coconut oil), pineapple juice (or orange juice), maple syrup, and vanilla.

3. Combine Dry and Wet Ingredients : Mix the wet ingredients into the dry ingredients until well combined.

4. Baking : Preheat the oven to the lowest temperature (between 180-200°F).

5. Pour the mixture onto trays.
6. Bake for 6 to 8 hours, ensuring the granola cooks evenly without burning. Adjust based on your oven settings

7. Storage : Once cooled, store the granola in an airtight container. The granola can last for several weeks when stored properly.

Notes : Barbara explains that granola can be enjoyed as breakfast or alternatively as a cereal, snack, or in various ways. The secret is to bake at a low temperature for an extended time (6-8 hours) so that the nutrients do not get lost, and it tastes the best. Adjust the sweetness and flavor by choosing different nuts or seeds. It doesn't last long because it's a favorite recipe. The cooking time is crucial, and experimenting with your oven settings is recommended.

Lunch

O'Neill repeatedly emphasizes having "a lunch like a queen." Barbara echoes this sentiment, indicating a relatively light lunch, akin to how a queen might dine. She often opts for a vegetable-based lunch.

Big Salad with Protein

Ingredients :

- Dark green leaves (e.g., spinach)
- Grated carrot
- Avocado slices
- Tomato slices
- Optional: Olives, bell peppers, or vegetables of choice
- Protein source (e.g., grilled chicken, chickpeas, lentils)
- Salad dressing: Olive oil, lemon juice, crushed garlic, salt, and herbs

Instructions :

Mix together a combination of green leaves, shredded carrot, creamy avocado, juicy tomato and any additional veggies you prefer in a bowl. Choose your protein source. Add it to the mix. In a jar combine olive oil, lemon juice, crushed garlic, salt and aromatic herbs to make a delicious dressing. Pour this dressing over the salad. Give it a toss to ensure everything is well coated.

Bean and Dressing Salad

Ingredients :

For the Dressing :
- Juice of one lemon
- 2 tablespoons olive oil
- 1 tablespoon tahini
- 1 clove garlic, crushed

For the Salad :
- 2 cups cooked cannellini beans (or other cooked beans of your choice), rinsed

Instructions :

1. Prepare the Dressing : In a small bowl, whisk together the lemon juice, olive oil, tahini, and crushed garlic.

2. Mix the Salad : In a larger bowl, add the rinsed cannellini beans or your chosen cooked beans.

3. Combine Dressing and Beans : Pour the prepared dressing over the beans. Gently toss to ensure that the beans are well coated with the dressing.

4. Adjust Seasoning : You can add more lemon juice, olive oil, or tahini based on your preference.

5. Chill (Optional) : You can refrigerate the salad for a while to let the flavors meld. This step is optional, and you can also serve it immediately.

Salsa Corn Dish

Ingredients :

- Fresh corn
- Cilantro
- Green onions
- Tomatoes
- Salt
- Limes
- Black beans

Instructions :

1. Mix the Fresh Ingredients : Mix fresh corn, chopped cilantro, sliced green onions, diced tomatoes, and black beans in a bowl.

2. Season : Add salt to taste, if needed. It could also be squeezed lime juice generously over the mixture for a zesty kick.

3. Harmonize Flavors : Mix all the ingredients thoroughly and allow the salsa to sit for a few minutes. This gives the flavors a chance to meld together, creating a delicious harmony.

4. Serve : Present your creation with class, be creative.

Notes : Barbara highlighted that this salsa corn dish aligns with a Weight Watchers recipe and is ideal for picnics and events, especially for those aiming for a lower-calorie meal. She emphasizes that anyone can adjust the quantities based on their taste preferences.

Egg Roll Bowl

Ingredients :

- Grass-fed ground beef (or ground turkey/chicken)
- Coleslaw mix
- Broccoli slaw
- Fish sauce
- Coconut aminos
- Soy sauce
- Honey
- Sriracha (optional)

Instructions :

Start by cooking up the ground beef in a pan until it's just right. Toss in the coleslaw mix and broccoli slaw to join the party. In a separate bowl, whip up a delightful sauce using fish sauce, coconut aminos, soy sauce, honey, and a dash of sriracha. Now, let the sauce rain down over the beef and veggies, giving them a tasty makeover. Stir it all up until everything's cozy and warmed through.

Notes : Barbara suggests that this egg roll bowl is a simple and quick lunch option, especially when we don't have a lot of time to prepare food.

Marinated Tofu

Ingredients :

- 1 block of firm or extra-firm tofu, pressed and cubed
- Juice of one lemon
- 3 tablespoons olive oil
- 2 cloves garlic, crushed
- 1 tablespoon grated ginger
- 1/2 teaspoon salt (adjust to taste)
- 1 tablespoon miso paste (optional, for added flavor)

Instructions :

11. Prepare the Tofu : Start by pressing the tofu to remove any water. Cut it into cubes according to your size.

12. Lets prepare the marinade : Take a bowl and whisk together lemon juice, olive oil, crushed garlic, grated ginger, salt and miso paste (if you have it). Make sure all the ingredients are well combined.

13. Time to marinate the tofu : Place the tofu cubes in a dish or a sealable plastic bag. Pour the marinade over them ensuring that each piece is thoroughly coated. You can refrigerate it for 30 minutes to let the flavors blend together or leave it longer for an even stronger flavor. If you plan on baking or grilling. If you want to bake the tofu, preheat your oven to heat (375°F/190°C) or get your grill ready.

14. Cooking instructions, for both methods :

   - Baking : Arrange the tofu cubes on a baking sheet and bake them in the preheated oven for 20-25 minutes until they turn golden brown.
   - Grilling :Thread the tofu cubes onto skewers. Grill them for approximately 10-15 minutes while turning occasionally until they acquire a beautiful charred appearance.

15. Serve : Serve the tofu in whichever way you prefer. Whether, on its own as an addition to a salad or as a versatile protein option in various dishes. If you'd like you can add a touch of freshness with some herbs. Sprinkle some sesame seeds on top, for added texture.

Mediterranean Roasted Vegetables with Olives

Ingredients :

- Baked sweet potato, cubed (leftover from the previous day)
- Roasted pumpkin, cubed (leftover from the previous day)
- 1 cup mixed olives (green and black), pitted
- 2 tablespoons olive oil
- 1 teaspoon dried oregano
- 1 teaspoon dried thyme
- Salt and pepper to taste
- Feta cheese for garnish (Optional)

Instructions :

1. Preheat the Oven : Preheat your oven to 400°F (200°C).

2. Prepare the Vegetables : If the sweet potato and pumpkin are not already cubed, cut them into bite-sized cubes.
3. Mix with Olives : In a large mixing bowl, combine the cubed sweet potato, pumpkin, and olives.

4. Season the Vegetables : Drizzle olive oil over the vegetables and olives. Sprinkle dried oregano, dried thyme, salt, and pepper. Toss the mixture until all the ingredients are well coated.

5. Roast in the Oven : Spread the vegetable and olive mixture evenly on a baking sheet. Roast in the preheated oven for about 20-25 minutes or until the vegetables are golden and slightly crispy at the edges.

6. Garnish with Feta : Crumble feta cheese can be added over the roasted vegetables just before serving for added flavor. (Optional)

7. Serve : Transfer the roasted vegetables and olives to a serving dish. This dish can be served warm or at room temperature.

Notes : This Mediterranean Roasted Vegetable dish makes for a flavorful and nutritious option with the sweetness of sweet potato and pumpkin complemented by the savory olives and herbs.

Nutrient-Rich Harmony Bowl

Ingredients :

- 1 cup cooked legumes of your choice (e.g., chickpeas, lentils, black beans)
- 10 mixed nuts (e.g., almonds, walnuts, pistachios)
- 1/4 cup mixed seeds (e.g., pumpkin seeds, sunflower seeds, chia seeds)
- Mixed vegetables (e.g., cherry tomatoes, cucumber, bell peppers)
- Fresh herbs (e.g., parsley, cilantro) for garnish
- 2 tablespoons olive oil
- 1 tablespoon balsamic vinegar
- 1 teaspoon Dijon mustard
- Salt and pepper to taste

Instructions :

1. Prepare Legumes : Cook legumes according to package instructions or use canned legumes, drained and rinsed.

2. Prepare Nuts and Seeds : Mix 10 nuts of your choice with 1/4 cup mixed seeds in a small bowl.

3. Chop Vegetables : Chop mixed vegetables into bite-sized pieces.

4. Assemble the Bowl : Combine cooked legumes, mixed nuts, seeds, and chopped vegetables in a large bowl.

5. Prepare Dressing : Whisk together olive oil, balsamic vinegar, Dijon mustard, salt, and pepper to create the dressing.
6. Drizzle Dressing and Toss : Drizzle the dressing over the mixture and gently toss until well coated.

7. Garnish : Garnish with fresh herbs for added flavor and freshness.

    Serve : Divide into serving bowls and enjoy the wholesome Legumes, Nuts, and Seeds Bowl.

Notes : This lunch option provides a balance of protein, healthy fats, and fiber from the legumes, nuts, and seeds.

Dinner

She suggests preparing soup for dinner, emphasizing simplicity, and avoiding foods that cause blood sugar levels to spike. However, as mentioned earlier, she also includes different other options in her diet for dinner, when she has dinner.

Chilled Cucumber and Mint Soup

Ingredients:

- 2 large cucumbers, peeled and diced
- 1/4 cup fresh mint leaves, plus extra for garnish
- 1 clove garlic, minced
- 1 tablespoon lemon juice
- Salt and pepper to taste

Instructions:

1. Blend Ingredients : In a blender, combine diced cucumbers, mint leaves, minced garlic, and lemon juice.

2. Blend Until Smooth : Blend until the mixture is smooth and creamy.

3. Season : Add salt and pepper to taste. Adjust the seasoning as needed.

4. Chill : Transfer the soup to a bowl and refrigerate for at least 1-2 hours to chill.

5. Serve : Ladle the chilled cucumber and mint soup into bowls. Drizzle with a bit of olive oil and garnish with extra mint leaves.

Notes : Barbara rarely consumes dinner, but when she does, one of her most frequently enjoyed meals is soup. As soup is highly subjective, feel free to modify the recipe as you like.

Avocado and Tomato Crackers

Ingredients:

- Whole-grain crackers
- 1 ripe avocado, sliced
- Cherry tomatoes, halved
- Fresh basil leaves
- Lemon juice
- Salt

Instructions:

1. <u>Prepare Crackers:</u> Place whole-grain crackers on a serving plate.

2. <u>Add Avocado Slices:</u> Place thin slices of ripe avocado on each cracker.

3. <u>Top with Tomatoes and Basil:</u> Add a halved cherry tomato on each cracker and garnish with fresh basil leaves.

4. <u>Drizzle with Lemon Juice:</u> Squeeze fresh lemon juice over the avocado and tomatoes.

5. <u>Serve:</u> Arrange the crackers on a plate and serve immediately.

Notes: Earlier in the book, it has been mentioned that Barbara doesn't have dinner often. However, when she does, she frequently opts for the crackers and avocado meal due to its lightness.

Vegetable Variety with Pesto Sauce

Ingredients:

- Baked beetroot and sweet potatoes
- Green beans
- Pesto sauce (homemade or store-bought)

Instructions:

Start by preheating the oven. Bake the beetroot and sweet potatoes until they are tender. In the meantime steam the beans until they are cooked but still have a crispness to them. Once everything is ready, arrange the vegetables and green beans on a plate. Finish it off by drizzling some pesto sauce over them. Now you can sit down. Enjoy a dinner that's not only tasty but also packed with nutrients.

Melon Salad

Ingredients:

- ❖ 2 cups diced melon (choose your favorite variety, such as cantaloupe or honeydew)
- ❖ Fresh mint leaves for garnish (optional)
- ❖ A squeeze of fresh lime or lemon juice (optional)

Instructions:

1. <u>Prepare the Melon:</u> Wash and peel the melon, removing seeds if necessary. Cut it into bite-sized cubes.

2. <u>Assemble the Salad :</u> Place the diced melon in a serving bowl.

- Garnish (Optional) : If you like, you can add a few fresh mint leaves for extra freshness and color.
- Add Citrus Squeeze (Optional) : For a burst of citrus flavor, squeeze a bit of fresh lime or lemon juice over the melon. This step is optional but can enhance the overall taste.
- Toss Gently (Optional) : If you'd like, you can gently toss the melon to distribute the citrus juice and mint.
- Chill (Optional) : You can refrigerate the melon salad for a short time if you prefer it chilled, but it's delicious served immediately as well.

3. <u>Serve :</u> Serve in individual bowls or as a light and refreshing side dish.

Notes : This Melon Salad is incredibly simple and Barbara suggests it, indicating it for a perfect light meal in the evening.

Snacks and dessert

Despite not consuming dessert or snacks on a daily basis, Barbara, in her lectures, guides us on how to make snacks, desserts, or extras to include in our meals. In this section, a few are mentioned:

Black Currant and Apple Jam

Ingredients :

- ❖ Dried black currants
- ❖ Apple and black carrot juice (no added sugar)

Instructions :

1. Prepare the Juice : In a saucepan, pour the apple and black carrot juice. Ensure that the juice has no added sugar for a healthier option.

2. Add Dried Black Currants : Measure the desired amount of dried black currants and add them to the saucepan with the juice. The quantity of currants can be adjusted based on your preference for sweetness and texture.

3. Heat the Mixture : Place the saucepan over medium heat and bring the juice and black currants to a gentle boil.

4. Boil gently and Infuse : Reduce the heat to a simmer and let the mixture cook for a while, allowing the dried black currants to absorb the flavors from the juice. Stir occasionally to ensure even distribution of ingredients.

5. Test for Consistency : To check the consistency, place a small amount of the jam on a cold plate. Run your finger through it; if it wrinkles and holds its shape, the jam is ready.

6. Cool and Store : Remove the saucepan from heat and let the jam cool to room temperature. Once cooled, transfer it to sterilized jars and store in the refrigerator.

Notes : Barbara mentions making this jam for her children and highlights that it doesn't last as long as traditional sugar jams.

Pear Cream

Ingredients :

- Brazil nuts or cashews
- Tinned pears in natural juice
- Coconut cream (optional)
- Vanilla essence

Instructions :

Blend Brazil nuts or cashews with tinned pears in natural juice. Optionally, add coconut cream for extra creaminess. Add vanilla essence for flavor.

Notes : Barbara suggests using the pear cream on various desserts and highlights its slightly sweet taste from the natural pear juice.

Carob Balls

Ingredients :

- Tahini
- Maple syrup or honey
- Coconut cream or coconut oil
- Ground nuts
- Carob powder

Instructions :

Mix tahini, maple syrup or honey, coconut cream or oil, ground nuts, and carob powder. Then, form the mixture into balls. Lastly, freeze the balls.

Notes : Barbara mentions rolling the balls in coconut oil or cream and then freezing them. Carob is described as having a naturally sweet flavor.

Banana Cake

Ingredients :

- Ripe bananas
- Coconut oil
- Olive oil
- Sweetener (Palm sugar or maple syrup)
- White and wholemeal spelled flour
- Walnuts
- Sultanas (Raisins)
- Baking powder

Instructions:

Blend ripe bananas, coconut oil, olive oil, sweetener, and a mix of white and wholemeal spelt flour. Fold in walnuts and sultanas. Bake until done.

Notes: Barbara emphasizes the use of bananas and oils for a lighter cake. Also, she mentions avoiding milk or water in the recipe.

Waffle Cake

Ingredients:

- Soaked chickpeas
- Raw millet
- Water
- Salt
- Fruit jam
- Pear cream

Instructions:

lend soaked chickpeas, raw millet, water, and salt to make waffle batter. Cook waffles in a waffle iron. Lastly, layer waffles with fruit jam and pear cream.

Notes: Barbara explains that the waffle cake is served with layers of fruit jam and pear cream, creating a unique and delicious dessert.

Apple Pie

Ingredients:

- Apples
- Sultanas (Raisins)
- Spelled flour

- Olive oil
- Water
- Pinch of salt

Instructions:

Cook apples in water until soft, then sprinkle with sultanas. Prepare pastry using spelt flour, olive oil, water, and salt. Bake with a bottom crust, add the softened apples, and cover with the top crust. Continue baking until golden brown.

Notes: Barbara enjoys apple pie once a week, and it's important to note that no sweeteners are added to the recipe. The pastry is crafted with spelt flour, and Barbara emphasizes the use of low-glycemic index ingredients.

Pumpkin Pie

Ingredients:

- Pumpkin
- Dates
- Coconut cream
- Coriander
- Cinnamon
- Grated lemon rind
- Spelled flour (for crust)

Instructions:

To make this delicious pumpkin pie, start by cooking the pumpkin with dates until it's soft. Then, add coconut cream, coriander, cinnamon, and grated lemon rind to enhance the flavor. After that, blend the mixture until it reaches a smooth consistency. For the crust, use spelled flour and bake the entire pie until it achieves a golden brown perfection. This simple yet flavorful recipe promises a delightful pumpkin pie experience.

Notes: Barbara highlights the use of coconut cream for creaminess and the addition of spices for flavor.

Tea

Barbara has frequently mentioned the phrase "Tea, like a pauper" indicating her belief in savoring tea in a way without customs or costly ingredients. Despite being someone who regularly enjoys tea Barbara cautions against consuming caffeine.

Liver Cleansing Tea Recipe

Ingredients:

- 1 scoop of liver cleanse mixture (Dandelion root, Licorice root, Gentian root, Milk Thistle, Goldenseal)
- 2 cups of water

Instructions:

Start by heating up water in a stainless steel pot until it reaches a simmer. Next add one teaspoon of the mixture into the pot, cover it with a lid and keep it simmering for 15 minutes.

Notes: Barbara explains that this tea, which helps cleanse the liver, contains elements such as Dandelion root and Milk Thistle that are known for their ability to promote liver health and detoxification. It is suggested to drink this tea in the morning along with a liver cleanse mixture as part of a complete detox regimen.

Herbal Bowel Support Tea Recipe

Ingredients:

- 1 teaspoon of herbal mixture (Dandelion root, Licorice root, Gentian root, and other herbs)
- 8 oz of water
- Honey for sweetness (Optional)

Instructions:

Begin by heating water in a stainless steel pot until it reaches a simmer. Then take one teaspoon of the blend. Add it to the pot. Turn off the heat. Allow the mixture to cool down. If desired you can add honey for some sweetness. Finally strain the liquid using a strainer. Make it a habit to drink this tea regularly particularly when dealing with any bowel related concerns.

Notes: This herbal blend is designed to be gentle, on the system. It helps support bowel movements and promotes gut health. It can be an addition to probiotics, for maintaining a gut and can also aid in relieving constipation thus promoting
overall digestive wellness.

UNLOCKING NATURE'S PHARMACY

The Hidden Trove of Forbidden Remedies Big Pharma Doesn't Want You to Discover

In a world where the pharmaceutical giants hold sway, the simple, profound truth often escapes our notice : "THE BODY CAN HEAL ITSELF." Despite the overwhelming evidence supporting natural healing methods, these truths are frequently obscured, if not outright suppressed, by those who profit from the sale of synthetic medications. It's no secret that there exists a vast array of natural remedies potent enough to mitigate, if not outright cure, many of the ailments for which modern medicine too often prescribes chemical solutions.

The pharmaceutical companies do not want you to know this!

Our reliance on manufactured pharmaceuticals comes at a cost, not just to our wallets but to our health and well-being. Nature offers a pharmacy of its own, rich with healing agents that have been used effectively for thousands of years. These natural remedies can empower the body to heal itself, often without the side effects associated with drugs.

Note: This book could be censored at any moment, buy it without thinking, don't say we didn't warn you...

Below, we present 25 recipes for "Herbal Antibiotics" — each with detailed descriptions of their uses. These are not mere alternatives but primary go-to solutions that align with our body's natural defenses, offering potent cures to various ailments and infections. Through these recipes, we aim to provide you with the knowledge to harness these powerful, natural solutions and thus take a stand against the monopolistic practices of the pharmaceutical industry.

25 recipes for Herbal Antibiotics

Garlic Tincture

Ingredients:

- Fresh garlic
- Vodka
- Brandy

Preparation:

1. Crush garlic cloves

2. Submerge in alcohol

3. Let sit for 2-4 weeks

4. Strain

Uses:

- Natural antibiotic
- Effective against bacteria and viruses.

Echinacea Extract

Ingredients:

- Echinacea roots and leaves

- Alcohol or glycerin.

Preparation :

1. Chop roots and leaves

2. Cover with alcohol

3. Let steep for 4-6 weeks

4. Strain.

Uses :

- Boosts the immune system and fights infections.

Goldenseal Tincture

Ingredients :

- Dried goldenseal root
- Alcohol

Preparation :

1. Powder root

2. Soak in alcohol for 4 weeks

3. Strain.

Uses :

- Antibacterial and antifungal
- Good for respiratory and digestive infections.

Oregano Oil Capsules

Ingredients :

- Oregano essential oil
- Olive oil
- Gelatin capsules

Preparation :

1. Mix oregano oil with olive oil

2. Fill capsules.

Uses :

- Antimicrobial properties
- Effective against bacteria and viruses.

Thyme Syrup

Ingredients :

- Fresh thyme
- Water
- Honey

Preparation :

1. Boil thyme in water

2. Strain

3. Add honey

4. Simmer until syrupy.

Uses :

- Treats respiratory infections and coughs.

Ginger and Honey Paste

Ingredients :

- Fresh ginger
- Honey.

Preparation :

1. Grate ginger

2. Mix with honey

3. Store in a jar.

Uses:

- Soothes sore throats and boosts immunity.

Sage Mouthwash

Ingredients:

- Sage leaves
- Water

Preparation:

1. Boil sage in water

2. Strain

3. Use as a gargle.

Uses:

- Boil sage in water

- Strain

- Use as a gargle.

Lavender Infused Oil

Ingredients:

- Lavender flowers
- Carrier oil

Preparation:

1. Fill jar with flowers

2. Cover with oil

3. Let sit for 3-6 weeks

4. Strain.

Uses:

- Antibacterial
- Good for skin infections and relaxation

Cayenne Pepper Salve

Ingredients:

- Cayenne pepper
- Olive oil
- Beeswax

Preparation:

1. Infuse oil with cayenne

2. Melt in beeswax

3. Cool into a salve.

Uses:

- Anti-inflammatory and antibacterial
- Good for wounds.

Turmeric and Black Pepper Capsules

Ingredients:

- Turmeric powder

- Ground black pepper
- Capsules

Preparation :

1. Mix turmeric with black pepper

2. Fill capsules.

Uses :

- Anti-inflammatory
- Antioxidant
- Antibacterial.

Clove Toothache Drops

Ingredients :

- Clove oil
- Olive oil

Preparation :

1. Mix oils

2. Apply directly to gums or tooth

Uses :

- Natural anesthetic and antibacterial
- Relieves tooth pain

Aloe Vera and Tea Tree Gel

Ingredients :

- Aloe vera gel
- Tea tree oil

Preparation :

1. Mix aloe vera with a few drops of tea tree oil

2. Apply to skin

Uses:

- Antibacterial and antifungal
- Great for skin infections and acne

Calendula Wound Salve

Ingredients:

- Calendula flowers
- Coconut oil
- Beeswax

Preparation:

1. Infuse oil with flowers

2. Melt with beeswax

3. Pour into containers

Uses:

- Antiseptic and antibacterial
- Promotes wound healing.

Peppermint Cooling Spray

Ingredients:

- Peppermint essential oil
- Water

Preparation:

1. Mix oil with water in a spray bottle

Uses:

- Antimicrobial and soothing
- Good for sunburn and hot skin

Lemon Balm Herpes Cream

Ingredients:

- Lemon balm
- Olive oil
- Beeswax

Preparation:

1. Infuse oil with lemon balm

2. Blend with beeswax and cool

Uses:

- Antiviral
- Particularly effective against herpes simplex virus

Cinnamon Lip Balm

Ingredients:

- Cinnamon oil
- Coconut oil
- Beeswax

Preparation:

1. Melt beeswax

2. Mix in oils

3. Pour into lip balm tubes

Uses:

- Antibacterial
- Prevents and treats lip infections

Basil Leaf Poultice

Ingredients:

- Fresh basil leaves.

Preparation:

1. Crush leaves

2. Apply directly to the affected area.

Uses:

- Antibacterial
- Good for insect **bites and stings**

Neem Leaf Paste

Ingredients:

- Neem leaves
- Water

Preparation:

1. Grind leaves with water to form a pasteapply to skin

Uses:

- Antifungal and antibacterial
- Treats skin disorders

Juniper Berry Diuretic Tea

Ingredients:

- Juniper berries
- Water

Preparation:

1. Crush berries

2. Steep in hot water

3. Strain

Uses:

- Antibacterial
- Aids kidney and urinary tract health

Horseradish Sinus Remedy

Ingredients:

- Horseradish root
- Vinegar

Preparation:

1. Grate root

2. Cover with vinegar

3. Let sit

4. Strain

Uses:

- Antibiotic properties
- Clears sinuses

Elderberry Immune Booster

Ingredients:

- Elderberries
- Water
- Honey

Preparation:

1. Simmer berries in water

2. Mash

3. Strain

4. Add honey

Uses:

- Antiviral
- Boosts immunity
- Especially during cold and flu season

Yarrow Styptic Powder

Ingredients :

- Dried yarrow flowers

Preparation :

1. Grind flowers into a fine powder

Uses :

- Antibacterial
- Stops bleeding from cuts and scrapes

Plantain Leaf Skin Soother

Ingredients :

- Plantain leaves

Preparation :

1. Crush or blend leaves

2. Apply as a poultice or rinse

Uses :

- Antibacterial and anti-inflammatory
- Treats skin irritations

Marshmallow Root Cough Syrup

Ingredients:

- Marshmallow root
- Water
- Honey

Preparation:

1. Simmer root in water
2. Strain

3. Mix with honey

Uses:

- Soothes sore throats and relieves coughs

Chickweed Ointment

Ingredients:

- Chickweed
- Olive oil
- Beeswax

Preparation:

1. Infuse chickweed in olive oil

2. Strain

3. Melt with beeswax

4. Cool into ointment.

Uses:

- Anti-inflammatory and antiseptic
- Good for eczema and other skin conditions

Each of these remedies offers a natural alternative to synthetic antibiotics, leveraging the intrinsic antibacterial and antiviral properties of herbs and natural substances to treat and prevent various health issues.

25 Remedies and Recipes for Skin and Hair Care

Below, we unveil an array of recipes designed for skin and hair care — each enriched with detailed explanations of their uses. These are not just supplementary choices; they are essential tools that resonate with the natural healing mechanisms of our bodies, providing effective treatments for a variety of skin and hair conditions. With these recipes, we aim to equip you with the means to tap into these potent, natural solutions, empowering you to reclaim your health from the profit-driven motives of the pharmaceutical industry. By integrating these remedies into your daily routine, you take a crucial step towards holistic wellness, steering clear of the synthetic compounds that dominate the market today.

Aloe Vera Gel Moisturizer

Ingredients:

- Fresh aloe vera gel

Preparation:

1. Extract gel from leaves

2. Apply directly to skin

Uses:

- Deep conditions hair
- Adds shine and strength

Coconut Oil Hair Mask

Ingredients:

- Virgin coconut oil

Preparation:

1. Warm oil

2. Apply to hair

3. Leave for 1 hour

4. Wash out

Uses :

- Deep conditions hair
- Adds shine and strength

Tea Tree Oil Acne Treatment

Ingredients :

- Tea tree oil
- Water

Preparation :

1. Dilute tea tree oil with water

2. Apply with a cotton ball to affected areas

Uses :

- Natural antibacterial
- Treats acne

Oatmeal Bath Soak

Ingredients :

- Ground oatmeal

Preparation :

1. Add to bathwater

2. Soak for 15-20 minutes

Uses :

- Soothes itchy
- Irritated skin

Rose Water Toner

Ingredients :

- Rose petals
- Water

Preparation :

Boil petals in water, strain, cool, and use as a facial toner.

Uses :

- Tones and refreshes skin
- Maintains pH balance.

Avocado Hair Conditioner

Ingredients :

- Riocado
- Olive oil

Preparation :

1. Mash avocado

2. Mix with olive oil

3. Apply to hair

4. Rinse after 20 minutes.

Uses :

- Nourishes the scalp and promotes hair growth..

Chamomile Face Wash

Ingredients:

- Chamomile tea

Preparation:

1. Brew tea

2. Cool

3. Use as a gentle face wash

Uses:

- Calms skin and reduces redness

Lavender Sleep Mask

Ingredients:

- Lavender essential oil
- aloe vera gel

Preparation:

1. Mix and apply to face before bed

Uses:

- Promotes relaxation and soothes skin overnight

Coffee Scrub for Cellulite

Ingredients:

- Ground coffee
- Coconut oil

Preparation :

1. Mix
2. Scrub on damp skin

3. Rinse

Uses :

- Exfoliates and increases blood flow to reduce cellulite

Apple Cider Vinegar Hair Rinse

Ingredients :

- Apple cider vinegar,
- Water

Preparation :

1. Mix

2. Use as a final rinse after shampooing

Uses :

- Cleanses scalp
- Restores hair shine.

Honey Face Mask

Ingredients :

- Apple cider vinegar
- Water

Preparation :

1. Apply directly to face

2. Leave for 20 minutes

3. Rinse off

Uses:

- Moisturizes and fights skin infections

Argan Oil Hair Serum

Ingredients:

- Argan oil

Preparation:

1. Apply a few drops to damp or dry hair ends

Uses:

- Smoothens hair
- Reduces frizz

Cucumber Eye Pads

Ingredients:

- Fresh cucumber

Preparation:

1. Slice thinly

2. Place over eyes for 15 minutes

Uses:

- Reduces under-eye puffiness and dark circles

Shea Butter Body Cream

Ingredients :

- Shea butter
- Coconut oil
- Essential oil of choice

Preparation :

1. Melt shea butter and coconut oil

2. Add essential oil

3. Cool until solid

Uses :

- Intensely moisturizes and heals dry skin

Turmeric Brightening Paste

Ingredients :

- Turmeric powder
- Lemon juice
- Honey

Preparation :

1. Mix into a paste

2. Apply to face

3. Wash off after 15 minutes

Uses :

- Reduces dark spots and scars

Peppermint Scalp Stimulator

Ingredients:

- Peppermint oil
- Water

Preparation:

1. Dilute peppermint oil with water

2. Massage into scalp

Uses:

- Promotes hair growth by stimulating the scalp

Bentonite Clay Mask

Ingredients:

- Bentonite clay
- Water

Preparation:

1. Mix to form a paste

2. Apply to skin

3. Rinse after drying.

Uses:

- Detoxifies skin
- tightens and cleans pores

Jojoba Oil Cuticle Cream

Ingredients:

- Jojoba oil
- Beeswax

Preparation :

1. Melt beeswax

2. mix in jojoba oil

3. cool in a small jar

Uses :

- Moisturizes and nourishes nail cuticles

Almond Oil Stretch Mark Reducer

Ingredients :

- Sweet almond oil

Preparation :

1. Massage into stretch marks daily

Uses :

- Reduces the appearance of stretch marks

Lemon Salt Foot Scrub

Ingredients :

- Sea salt
- Lemon juice
- Olive oil

Preparation :

1. Mix

2. Scrub feet

3. Rinse

Uses:

- Exfoliates and refreshes tired feet

Rice Water Hair Rinse

Ingredients:

- Rice
- Water

Preparation:

1. Soak rice in water

2. Strain

3. Use rinse on hair after shampooing.

Uses:

- Strengthens hair and adds shine

Green Tea Toner

Ingredients:

- Green tea

Preparation:

1. Brew strong tea

2. Cool

3. Apply to face with a cotton ball

Uses:

- Reduces skin inflammation and acne

Mango Body Butter

Ingredients:

- Mango butter
- Coconut oil
- Vitamin E oil

Preparation:

1. Melt ingredients together

2. Cool until solid

Uses:

- Reduces skin inflammation and acne

Basil and Mint Pore Tightening Mask

Ingredients:

- Basil leaves
- Mint leaves
- Honey

Preparation:

1. Blend leaves with honey

2. Apply to face

3. Rinse off after 10 minutes

Uses:

- Tightens pores and refreshes the skin

Carrot and Coconut Oil Anti-Aging Facial Serum

Ingredients:

- Carrot seed oil
- Coconut oil

Preparation :

1. Mix oils

2. Apply to face before bed

Uses :

- Moisturizes skin
- Rich in vitamins for anti-aging

These recipes provide a variety of options for both everyday care and specific skin and hair concerns, utilizing natural ingredients known for their beneficial properties without the harsh chemicals found in many commercial products.

25 Remedies and Recipes for Enhancing Digestive Health

Here, we present a carefully curated collection of remedies and recipes designed to support and enhance digestive health using natural ingredients and herbal solutions. These selections go beyond mere supplements; they are fundamental treatments that work in harmony with your body's natural processes, promoting optimal digestive function. With these recipes, our goal is to empower you with the tools to harness the healing power of nature, enabling you to counter the pervasive influence of the pharmaceutical industry with effective, natural alternatives. Embrace these solutions to nurture your digestive health through the gentle efficacy of nature's own provisions.

Peppermint Tea

Ingredients :

- Peppermint leaves
- Hot water

Preparation :

1. Steep peppermint leaves in hot water for 5-10 minutes

2. Strain and drink

Uses :

- Eases digestive discomfort and reduces bloating

Ginger Digestive Chews

Ingredients :

* Fresh ginger
* Honey
* Lemon juice

Preparation :

1. Juice ginger

2. Mix with honey and lemon juice

3. Simmer until thick

4. Then cool and cut into small chewable pieces

Uses :

* Relieves nausea and improves digestion

Fennel Seed Tea

Ingredients :

* Fennel seeds
* Hot water

Preparation :

1. Crush fennel seeds

2. Steep in hot water for 5-10 minutes

3. Strain and drink

Uses :

* Reduces gas and bloating
* Stimulates digestion

Probiotic Yogurt Parfait

Ingredients:

- Plain probiotic yogurt

- Fresh berries

- Granola

Preparation:

1. Layer yogurt

2. Berries

3. Granola in a glass and enjoy

Uses:

- Supports gut health with live beneficial bacteria

Apple Cider Vinegar Tonic

Ingredients:

- Apple cider vinegar
- Warm water
- Honey

Preparation:

1. Mix a tablespoon of apple cider vinegar and honey in a cup of warm

Uses:

- Balances stomach pH and aids in digestion

Dandelion Root Tea

Ingredients:

- Dandelion root
- Hot water

Preparation :

2. Simmer dandelion root in water for 10 minutes

3. Strain and drink

Uses :

- Stimulates liver function and aids digestion

Lemon and Ginger Morning Elixir

Ingredients :

- Lemon juice
- Fresh ginger
- Hot water

Preparation :

1. Mix lemon juice and grated ginger in hot water

2. Drink on an empty stomach.

Uses :

- Kickstarts digestion and detoxifies

Banana and Oat Digestive Smoothie

Ingredients :

- Ripe banana
- Rolled oats
- Almond milk
- Honey

Preparation :

1. Blend all ingredients until smooth

Uses:

- Soothes the digestive tract and provides fiber

Cumin Digestive Aid

Ingredients:

- Cumin seeds
- Hot water

Preparation:

1. Boil cumin seeds in water for a few minutes

2. Strain and drink the water after meals

Uses:

- Stimulates digestive enzymes

Herbal Bitters

Ingredients:

- Dandelion root
- Gentian root
- Orange peel
- Alcohol

Preparation:

1. Macerate the herbs in alcohol for 4 weeks

2. Strain and use a few drops before meals

Uses:

- Stimulate bile production and improve digestion

Aloe Vera Juice

Ingredients :

- Fresh aloe vera gel
- Water

Preparation :

1. Blend aloe gel with water

2. Strain

3. Drink

Uses :

- Soothes the lining of the stomach and intestines

Chamomile Soothing Tea

Ingredients :

- Chamomile flowers
- Hot water

Preparation :

1. Steep chamomile flowers in hot water

2. Strain

3. Drink at bedtime

Uses :

- Reduces stomach discomfort and relaxes the digestive tract

Papaya Enzyme Salad

Ingredients :

- Fresh papaya
- Lime juice

- Honey

Preparation :

1. Cube papaya

2. Drizzle with lime juice and honey

3. Serve chilled

Uses :

- Contains natural enzymes that aid in protein digestion

Beet and Ginger Detox Juice

Ingredients :

- Beetroot
- Ginger
- Apple
- Carrot

Preparation :

1. Juice all ingredients

2. Drink fresh

Uses :

- Cleanses the liver and improves digestion

Sauerkraut

Ingredients :

- Cabbage
- Salt

Preparation :

1. Shred cabbage

2. Mix with salt

3. Pack into airtight jars

4. Let ferment for several weeks

Uses:

- Provides probiotics to aid digestion

Turmeric Milk

Ingredients:

- Turmeric powder
- Warm milk
- Honey

Preparation:

1. Mix turmeric in warm milk

2. Add honey to taste

3. Drink before bed

Uses:

- Anti-inflammatory
- Soothes digestive inflammation

Kombucha

Ingredients:

- Tea
- Sugar
- SCOBY (symbiotic culture of bacteria and yeast)

Preparation:

1. Brew tea

2. Add sugar, coo

3. Add SCOBY

4. Frment for 7-14 days

5. Then bottle

Uses :

- Probiotic-rich drink for gut health

Mint Refreshing Infusion

Ingredients :

- Fresh mint leaves
- Hot water

Preparation :

1. Steep mint leaves in hot water

2. Strain

3. Drink after meals

Uses :

- Relieves indigestion and cools the stomach

Licorice Root Digestive Tea

Ingredients :

- Licorice root
- Hot water

Preparation :

1. Simmer licorice root in hot water

2. Strain

3. Drink twice daily

Uses :

- Soothes gastrointestinal tissues and relieves acid reflux

Flaxseed Digestive Muffins

Ingredients :

- Ground flaxseeds
- Whole wheat flour
- Baking powder
- Eggs
- Milk

Preparation :

1. Mix ingredients

2. Pour into muffin tins

3. Bake at 350°F for 20 minutes

Uses :

- Provides fiber to aid digestion

Caraway Digestive Cookies

Ingredients :

- Caraway seeds
- Flour
- Butter
- Sugar

Preparation :

1. Mix ingredients

2. Form cookies

3. Bake until golden

Uses :

- Caraway seeds relieve bloating and gas

Basil and Lime Digestive Aid

Ingredients:

- Fresh basil
- Lime zest
- Olive oil

Preparation:

1. Blend ingredients

2. Use as a dressing or marinade

Uses:

- Stimulates digestion and adds flavor to meals

Pineapple Digestive Enzyme Smoothie

Ingredients:

- Fresh pineapple
- Yogurt
- Honey

Preparation:

1. Blend ingredients

2. Use as a dressing or marinade

Uses:

- Bromelain in pineapple helps break down proteins

Warm Lemon Water

Ingredients :

- Fresh lemon juice
- Warm water

Preparation :

1. Squeeze lemon into warm water

2. Drink first thing in the morning

Uses :

- Stimulates digestion and detoxifies

Cardamom Pod Tea

Ingredients :

- Cardamom pods
- Hot water

Preparation :

1. Crush pods slightly

2. Steep in hot water

3. Strain and drink after meals

Uses :

- Relieves heartburn and soothes the stomach

These recipes are designed to provide natural and effective solutions for a variety of digestive issues, enhancing overall digestive health through the thoughtful use of beneficial herbs and ingredients.

15-Day Gut Cleanse Plan

Day	Morning	Midday	Evening	Notes
1	Warm Lemon Water	Peppermint Tea	Chamomile Soothing Tea	Begin the day by stimulating digestion with lemon water. Peppermint tea after lunch aids digestion. Chamomile tea at bedtime soothes the digestive tract.
2	Ginger Digestive Chews	Apple Cider Vinegar Tonic	Fennel Seed Tea	Ginger chews in the morning help reduce nausea and kickstart digestion. ACV tonic before lunch improves digestion. Fennel tea in the evening to reduce gas.
3	Aloe Vera Juice	Kombucha	Mint Refreshing Infusion	Aloe vera juice soothes the stomach lining. Drink kombucha at lunch for probiotics. Mint infusion after dinner aids digestion.
4	Turmeric Milk	Lemon and Ginger Morning Elixir	Licorice Root Digestive Tea	Turmeric milk reduces inflammation. Lemon and ginger elixir after breakfast. Licorice tea to relieve acid reflux at night.
5	Pineapple Digestive Enzyme Smoothie	Sauerkraut	Warm Lemon Water	Pineapple smoothie in the morning for enzymes. Sauerkraut with lunch for probiotics. Lemon water in the evening.

6	Dandelion Root Tea	Probiotic Yogurt Parfait	Cumin Digestive Aid	Dandelion tea to stimulate the liver. Yogurt parfait at lunch. Cumin water after dinner to aid digestion.
7	Cardamom Pod Tea	Beet and Ginger Detox Juice	Apple Cider Vinegar Tonic	Start with cardamom tea for heartburn. Beet juice at noon detoxifies. ACV tonic in the evening.
8	Banana and Oat Digestive Smoothie	Ginger Digestive Chews	Peppermint Tea	Banana smoothie for breakfast. Ginger chews before lunch. Peppermint tea at night.
9	Warm Lemon Water	Chamomile Face Wash	Herbal Bitters	Lemon water in the morning. Chamomile post-lunch for calming. Herbal bitters before dinner.
10	Aloe Vera Juice	Kombucha	Fennel Seed Tea	Aloe vera to start the day. Kombucha at lunch for gut health. Fennel tea in the evening.
11	Ginger and Honey Paste	Lemon and Ginger Morning Elixir	Mint Refreshing Infusion	Ginger and honey for morning anti-inflammatory benefits. Lemon and ginger elixir after lunch. Mint infusion at night.
12	Pineapple Digestive Enzyme Smoothie	Sauerkraut	Licorice Root Digestive Tea	Pineapple smoothie for enzymes. Sauerkraut at lunch for gut health. Licorice tea at bedtime.

13	Turmeric Milk	Apple Cider Vinegar Tonic	Chamomile Soothing Tea	Turmeric milk in the morning. ACV tonic before lunch. Chamomile tea to end the day.
14	Warm Lemon Water	Probiotic Yogurt Parfait	Cumin Digestive Aid	Lemon water to start. Yogurt parfait for lunch. Cumin digestive aid after dinner.
15	Dandelion Root Tea	Beet and Ginger Detox Juice	Peppermint Tea	Dandelion tea in the morning. Beet and ginger juice at noon. Peppermint tea at night to soothe the digestive tract.

25 Powerful Immune-Boosting Recipes and Remedies

Discover our collection of 25 dynamic recipes and remedies, each crafted to strengthen your immune system using nature's most potent ingredients. These powerful solutions harness the intrinsic health-promoting properties of natural elements to fortify your body's defenses. Embrace these transformative recipes and take control of your health, naturally.

Elderberry Syrup

Ingredients:

- Elderberries
- Water
- Honey
- Ginger

Preparation :

1. Simmer elderberries with water and ginger

2. Strain

3. Add honey

4. Bottle

Uses :

- Prevents and eases cold and flu symptoms

Turmeric and Black Pepper Tea

Ingredients :

- Turmeric powder
- Black pepper
- Lemon juice
- Hot water

Preparation :

1. Mix turmeric and black pepper in hot water

2. Add lemon juice
3. Drink daily.

Uses :

- Anti-inflammatory and boosts immunity.

Garlic and Honey Immune Tonic

Ingredients :

- Raw garlic
- Honey

Preparation :

1. Chop garlic

2. Mix with honey

3. Let sit for a few days

4. Consume a spoonful daily.

Uses:

- Antibacterial and antiviral properties

Ginger Lemonade

Ingredients:

- Fresh ginger
- Lemon juice
- Honey
- Water

Preparation:

1. Juice ginger

2. Mix with lemon juice and honey

3. Dilute with water

4. Serve chilled.

Uses:

- Boosts immune response and detoxifies the body.

Vitamin C Smoot

Ingredients:

- Oranges
- Strawberries
- Kiwi
- Almond milk

Preparation:

1. Blend all ingredients until smooth

2. Drink immediately

Uses :

- Rich in vitamin C for immune support

Green Tea and Honey

Ingredients :

- Green tea leaves
- Honey

Preparation :

1. Brew green tea

2. Add honey while warm

3. Drink twice daily

Uses :

- Antioxidants and antibacterial properties

Zinc-Rich Pumpkin Seeds Snack

Ingredients :

- Pumpkin seeds
- olive oil
- Sea salt

Preparation :

1. Roast pumpkin seeds with olive oil and salt

2. Snack regularly

Uses :

- Provides zinc which is crucial for immune function

Mushroom Broth Soup

Ingredients :

- Shiitake mushrooms
- Onions
- Garlic
- Vegetable broth

Preparation :

1. Simmer all ingredients

2. Strain or blend for a hearty soup

Uses :

- High in immune-boosting minerals and vitamins

Kombucha

Ingredients :

- Kombucha SCOBY
- Tea
- Sugar

Preparation :

1. Brew tea

2. Add sugar

3. Cool

4. Add SCOBY

5. Ferment

6. Bottle

Uses:

- Probiotic-rich for gut health and immunity

Spicy Cayenne Pepper Sauce

Ingredients:

- Cayenne peppers
- vinegar
- salt

Preparation:

1. Blend peppers with vinegar and salt

2. Boil

3. Bottle

Uses:

- Capsaicin boosts metabolism and immune defense

Carrot and Ginger Juice

Ingredients:

- Carrots
- Fresh ginger
- Apple

Preparation:

1. Juice all ingredients

2. Drink fresh

Uses:

- High in vitamins A and C for immune support.

Oregano Oil

Ingredients :

- Oregano leaves
- Olive oil

Preparation :

1. Infuse oregano in olive oil for several weeks

2. Strain

3. Use a few drops daily

Uses :

- Natural antibiotic properties

Probiotic Yogurt

Ingredients :

- Milk
- Probiotic yogurt cultures

Preparation :

1. Heat milk

2. Cool

3. Add cultures

4. Ferment

5. Refrigerate

Uses :

- Enhances gut flora linked to improved immunity

Beet and Citrus Salad

Ingredients :

- Beets
- Oranges
- Walnuts
- Feta cheese

Preparation :

1. Roast beets

2. Segment oranges

3. Combine with walnuts and feta,

4. Dress lightly.

Uses :

- Rich in immune-boosting antioxidants and vitamin C

Brazil Nut Selenium Boost

Ingredients :

- Brazil nuts

Preparation :

1. Consume a few Brazil nuts daily

Uses :

- High in selenium
- Which is crucial for immune function

Sweet Potato Fries

Ingredients :

- Sweet potatoes

- Olive oil
- Salt.

Preparation:

1. Slice sweet potatoes

2. Toss with oil and salt

3. Bake until crispy

Uses:

- High in vitamins A and C.

Bone Broth

Ingredients:

- Bones
- water
- vinegar
- vegetables

Preparation:

1. Simmer bones with vinegar and vegetables for 24-48 hours

2. Strain

3. Consume warm

Uses:

- Rich in minerals and collagen
- Supports immune health

Chia Seed Pudding

Ingredients:

- Chia seeds
- Almond milk
- Honey

Preparation :

1. Mix chia seeds with almond milk and honey

2. Let sit until thickened

3. Enjoy

Uses :

- High in omega-3 fatty acids and fiber

Almond and Spinach Smoothie

Ingredients :

- Spinach
- Almond butter
- Banana
- Almond milk

Preparation :

1. Blend all ingredients until smooth

Uses :

- Packed with vitamin E
- Magnesium
- Iron

Sunflower Seed Butter

Ingredients :

- Sunflower seeds
- Olive oil

Preparation :

1. Process sunflower seeds and oil until creamy, store in the fridge

Uses :

- High in vitamin E and zinc

Sauerkraut

Ingredients :

- Cabbage
- Salt

Preparation :

1. Ferment shredded cabbage with salt

2. Consume regularly

Uses :

- Probiotic-rich
- Supports gut and immune health

Watermelon Mint Salad

Ingredients :

- Watermelon
- Fresh mint
- Feta cheese

Preparation :

1. Cube watermelon

2. Chop mint

3. Mix with crumbled feta

Uses :

- Hydrating and rich in lycopene and vitamin C

Honey and Cinnamon Warm Drink

Ingredients :

- Honey
- Cinnamon
- Hot water

Preparation :

1. Mix honey and cinnamon in hot water

2. Drink before bed

Uses :

- Antibacterial and soothing

Lentil and Garlic Soup

Ingredients :

- Lentils
- Garlic
- Onion
- Carrots
- Vegetable broth

Preparation :

1. Cook all ingredients until lentils are tender

2. Blend if desired

Uses :

- High in protein and allicin
- Which is antimicrobial

Flaxseed and Blueberry Oatmeal

Ingredients :

- Rolled oats
- Faxseeds
- Blueberries

- Almond milk

Preparation :

1. Cook oats in almond milk

2. Stir in flaxseeds and blueberries before serving.

Uses :

- Rich in antioxidants and omega-3 fatty acids

These recipes not only contribute to overall health but specifically support and strengthen the immune system, incorporating key nutrients that are vital for maintaining a robust defense against illness.

25 Stress and Anxiety Relief Strategies

Explore 25 targeted exercises, remedies, and recipes designed to alleviate stress and anxiety. Each method utilizes calming techniques and ingredients to soothe your mind and enhance relaxation.

Lavender Essential Oil Diffusion

Method :

1. Add a few drops of lavender oil to a diffuser and use in your living or bedroom.

Uses :

- Reduces anxiety and improves sleep

Chamomile Tea

Ingredients :

- Chamomile flowers
- Hot water

Method:

1. Steep chamomile flowers in hot water for 5-10 minutes

2. Strain

3. Drink

Uses:

- Calms nerves and soothes the stomach

Progressive Muscle Relaxation

Method:

1. Tense each muscle group for five seconds then relax for 30 seconds; repeat throughout the body.

Uses:

- Relieves muscle tension caused by stress

Yoga

Method:

1. Practice yoga sequences such as Sun Salutation or guided yoga sessions focusing on deep breathing.

Uses:

- Reduces stress
- Enhances mood
- Improves physical health

Mindfulness Meditation

Method:

1. Sit in a quiet place

2. Focus on your breath

3. Observe your thoughts without judgment for 10-20 minutes.

Uses:

- Reduces stress and improves concentration

Peppermint Tea

Ingredients:

- Peppermint leaves
- Hot water

Preparation:

1. Steep peppermint leaves in hot water

2. Strain

3. Enjoy

Uses:

- Relieves headaches and improves mental clarity

Guided Imagery

Method:

1. Listen to guided imagery scripts that lead you through peaceful scenes to help calm your mind.

Uses:

- Reduces anxiety through visualization

Journaling

Method:

1. Write down your thoughts

2. Feelings

3. Worries for 10 minutes each day to help clear your mind.

Uses :

- Helps process thoughts and reduces anxiety

CBD Oil

Method :

1. Consume CBD oil as per the dosage recommended by health professionals

Uses :

- Reduces anxiety without psychoactive effects

Green Tea

Ingredients :

- Green tea leaves
- Hot water

Preparation :

1. Brew green tea leaves

2. Drink twice daily

Uses :

- Contains L-theanine which can help reduce stress

Warm Epsom Salt Bath

Method :

1. Use essential oils like sandalwood or bergamot during a massage to help relax your muscles and mind

Uses :

- Relieves muscle tension and calms the mind

Aromatherapy Massage

Method:

1. Use essential oils like sandalwood or bergamot during a massage to help relax your muscles and mind

Uses:

- Reduces stress and physical tension

Breathing Exercises

Method:

1. Practice deep breathing techniques such as the 4-7-8 method—inhale for 4 seconds

2. Hold for 7 seconds

3. Exhale for 8 seconds

Uses:

- Promotes relaxation and reduces anxiety

Valerian Root Tea

Ingredients:

- Valerian root
- Hot water

Preparation:

1. Steep valerian root in hot water

2. Strain

3. Drink before bedtime

Uses:

- Helps with relaxation and sleep

Banana and Almond Smoothie

Ingredients:

- Banana
- Almond butter
- Almond milk

Preparation:

1. Blend ingredients until smooth

2. Drink as needed

Uses:

- Provides magnesium and potassium
- Help relax muscles and nerves

Regular Exercise

Method:

1. Engage in 30 minutes of moderate exercise like walking

2. Cycling

3. Swimming most days of the week

Uses:

- Reduces stress hormones and increases endorphins

Omega-3 Supplements

Method:

1. Take an omega-3 supplement daily

Uses:

- Reduces inflammation and anxiety

Herbal Sleep Tonic

Ingredients:

- Lemon balm
- Passionflower
- Water

Preparation:

1. Simmer herbs in water

2. Strain

3. Drink before bedtime

Uses:

- Promotes restful sleep
- Which is crucial for managing stress

Forest Bathing

Method:

1. Spend time walking slowly through a forest

2. Focusing on the sounds

3. Smells

4. Sights.

Uses:

- Reduces stress through nature immersion

B Vitamins

Method :

1. Include a B-complex vitamin supplement in your daily regimen

Uses :

- Essential for energy and brain function, helps reduce stress

Dark Chocolate

Method :

1. Eat a small piece of dark chocolate (at least 70% cocoa) daily

Uses :

- Contains flavonoids that increase serotonin levels

Lemon Balm Tea

Ingredients :

- Lemon balm leaves
- Hot water

Preparation :

1. Steep lemon balm in hot water

2. Strain

3. Drink as needed

Uses :

- Reduces anxiety and promotes calmness

Acupuncture

Method :

- Visit a licensed acupuncturist for sessions focusing on anxiety relief.

Uses :

- Lowers blood pressure and reduces cortisol

Acupuncture

Method :

1. Listen to calming music genres like classica

2. Jazz

3. Soft pop during stressful times.

Uses :

- Lowers blood pressure and reduces cortisol

St. John's Wort

Method :

1. Take St. John's wort supplements as directed by a healthcare provider

Uses :

- Natural remedy for mild to moderate anxiety

These activities, remedies, and dietary suggestions are designed to help manage stress and anxiety naturally, promoting a more relaxed and healthier state of mind.

25 Natural Remedies for Chronic Conditions

Discover 25 natural remedies and recipes, each tailored to manage and alleviate symptoms associated with chronic conditions, enhancing your health naturally.

Turmeric and Ginger Anti-Inflammatory Drink

Ingredients :

- Turmeric root
- Ginger root
- Black pepper
- Honey
- Lemon
- Hot water

Preparation :

Simmer turmeric and ginger in water

1. Strain

2. Add lemon and Honey

3. Sprinkle with black pepper

Uses :

- Reduces inflammation associated with conditions like arthritis

Flaxseed Oil Supplement

Method :

1. Consume 1 tablespoon of flaxseed oil daily or add it to salads

Uses :

- Provides omega-3 fatty acids to reduce inflammation

Cinnamon and Honey Mix

Ingredients:

- Cinnamon powder

- Raw honey

Preparation:

1. Mix cinnamon with honey and consume a spoonful each morning

Uses:

- Helps control blood sugar levels in diabetes

Hawthorn Berry Heart Tonic

Ingredients:

- Hawthorn berries
- water
- honey

Preparation:

1. Simmer berries in water for 20 minutes

2. Strain

3. Add honey

4. Drink twice daily.

Uses:

- Supports cardiovascular health

Nettle Tea

Ingredients:

- Dried nettle leaves
- Hot water

Preparation :

1. Steep nettle leaves in hot water for 10 minutes

2. Strain

3. Drink.

Uses :

- Rich in nutrients and helps in detoxification
- Beneficial for arthritis and kidney health.

Cherry Juice for Gout

Ingredients :

- Fresh or concentrate cherry juice

Method :

1. Drink a glass of cherry juice daily

Uses :

- Reduces uric acid levels and inflammation

Nettle Tea

Ingredients :

- Licorice root
- hot water

Preparation :

1. Simmer licorice root in hot water

2. Strain

3. Drink as a tea

Uses :

- Soothes gastrointestinal issues and can aid in adrenal fatigue

Aloe Vera Juice for Digestive Health

Ingredients :

- Fresh aloe vera gel
- Water

Preparation :

1. Blend aloe vera gel with water

2. Strain

3. Drink daily

Uses :

- Helps with digestion and soothes the stomach lining

Garlic Cardiovascular Remedy

Ingredients :

- Fresh garlic

Method :

1. Consume a raw garlic clove daily or include it in meals

Uses :

- Lowers blood pressure and cholesterol levels

Peppermint Oil Capsules for IBS

Ingredients :

- Peppermint oil

- Empty capsules

Preparation :

1. Fill capsules with peppermint oil

2. Take before meals

Uses :

- Relieves symptoms of irritable bowel syndrome

Ginger Anti-Nausea Drink

Ingredients :

- Fresh ginger
- Hot water
- Honey

Preparation :

Simmer ginger in hot water

1. Strain

2. Add honey

3. Drink

Uses :

- Helps with nausea and digestion issues

Omega-3 Rich Smoothie

Ingredients :

- Flaxseeds
- Chia seeds

- Spinach
- Blueberries
- Almond milk

Preparation :

1. Blend all ingredients until smooth

Uses :

- Supports joint health and reduces inflammation

Basil and Eucalyptus Respiratory Rub

Ingredients :

- Basil oil
- Eucalyptus oil
- Coconut oil

Preparation :

1. Mix oils with coconut oil

2. Apply to chest and back.

Uses :

- Helps clear respiratory pathways, useful for asthma or chronic bronchitis

Apple Cider Vinegar for Acid Reflux

Ingredients :

- Dried sage leaves
- Hot water

Preparation :

1. Mix a tablespoon of apple cider vinegar with a glass of water

2. Drink before meals.

Uses :

- Balances stomach pH and reduces acid reflux

Sage Tea for Throat Health

Ingredients:

- Dried sage leaves
- Hot water

Preparation:

1. Steep sage in hot water

2. Strain

3. Drink warm

Uses:

- Soothes sore throats and inflammation
- Helpful for chronic throat conditions

Milk Thistle Liver Tonic

Ingredients:

- Milk thistle seeds
- Hot water.

Preparation:

1. Crush seeds

2. Steep in hot water

3. Strain

4. Dink

Uses:

- Supports liver health and detoxification

Beet and Carrot Liver Cleanse Juice

Ingredients:

- Beetroot
- Carrot
- Lemon
- Ginger

Preparation:

1. Juice all ingredients

2. Drink fresh daily

Uses:

- Detoxifies the liver and improves liver function.

Cranberry Urinary Health Drink

Ingredients:

- Unsweetened cranberry juice
- Water

Preparation:

1. Mix cranberry juice with water

2. Drink daily

Uses:

- Prevents urinary tract infections

Oatmeal and Banana - Anti-inflammatory Breakfast

Ingredients:

- Rolled oats
- Banana
- Turmeric
- Almond milk

Preparation:

1. Cook oats in almond milk

2. Add sliced banana and a dash of turmeric

Uses:

- Provides lasting energy and anti-inflammatory benefits

Lavender and Chamomile Sleep Aid

Ingredients:

- Lavender flowers
- Chamomile flowers
- Hot water

Preparation:

1. Steep both in hot water

2. Strain

3. Drink before bedtime

Uses:

- Promotes restful sleep
- Helpful for chronic insomnia

Bromelain Pineapple Enzyme

Ingredients:

- Fresh pineapple

Method:

1. Eat fresh pineapple

2. Particularly the core which is rich in bromelain.

Uses:

- Reduces inflammation and aids digestion
- Beneficial for arthritis

Moringa Leaf Powder for Diabetes

Ingredients:

- Moringa leaf powder

Method:

1. Add a teaspoon of moringa powder to smoothies or soups.

Uses:

- Helps regulate blood sugar levels.

Spirulina Energy Booster

Ingredients:

- Spirulina powder

Method:

1. Mix spirulina powder into a glass of water or smoothie

Uses:

- Increases energy and nutrient intake, supports immune system

Ashwagandha Stress Relief

Ingredients:

- Ashwagandha powder
- Warm milk or water

Preparation :

1. Mix ashwagandha powder with warm milk or water

2. drink before bed

Uses :

- Reduces stress and anxiety
- Supports adrenal health

Capsaicin Cream for Pain Relief

Ingredients :

- Capsaicin extract
- Unscented lotion or coconut oil

Preparation :

1. Mix capsaicin with lotion or oil

2. Apply to painful areas

Uses :

- Relieves joint and muscle pain
- Useful for conditions like arthritis

These natural remedies and recipes offer supportive care for various chronic conditions, helping to manage symptoms and improve overall health and wellness.

25 Detox and Cleansing Recipes

Discover 25 recipes focused on detoxification and cleansing, crafted to purify the body and boost liver and kidney function while promoting overall wellness. Embrace these rejuvenating concoctions for a healthier you.

Green Detox Smoothie

Ingredients :

- Spinach
- Kale
- Green apple

- Cucumber
- Celery
- Lemon juice
- Ginger

Preparation :

1. Blend all ingredients with water until smooth for a powerful detoxifying drink.

Lemon Ginger Detox Tea

Ingredients :

- Lemon
- Fresh ginger
- Hot water

Preparation :

1. Slice lemon and ginger

2. Steep in hot water

3. Drink warm to help cleanse the liver and aid digestion.

Beetroot and Carrot Juice

Ingredients :

- Beetroot
- Carrot
- Fresh ginger
- Apple

Preparation :

1. Juice all ingredients for a nutrient-rich drink that supports liver detoxification.

Apple Cider Vinegar Elixir

Ingredients:

- Apple cider vinegar
- Warm water
- Honey
- Lemon juice

Preparation:

1. Mix all ingredients and drink in the morning to kick-start digestion and cleanse the system.

Activated Charcoal Lemonade

Ingredients:

- Activated charcoal
- Lemon juice
- Honey
- Water

Preparation:

1. Combine all ingredients and drink to help remove toxins from the body

Cilantro Detox Juice

Ingredients:

- Activated charcoal
- Lemon juice
- Honey
- Water

Preparation:

1. Juice all ingredients to create a drink that helps chelate heavy metals from the body.

Turmeric Liver Flush

Ingredients :

- Turmeric
- Lemon juice
- Olive oil
- Black pepper

Preparation :

1. Blend turmeric with lemon juice and olive oil

2. Sprinkle with black pepper and consume before bed to support liver detox.

Dandelion Root Tea

Ingredients :

- Dandelion root
- Hot water

Preparation :

1. Steep dandelion root in hot water

2. Strain and drink to support liver and kidney function.

Watermelon Mint Detox Water

Ingredients :

- Fresh watermelon
- Mint leaves
- Water

Preparation :

1. Mix watermelon cubes and mint leaves in water and infuse for a few hours to hydrate and detoxify.

Parsley Detox Smoothie

Ingredients :

- Fresh parsley
- Lemon juice
- Cucumber
- Apple
- Celery

Preparation :

1. Blend all ingredients with water for a detoxifying green smoothie

Chia Seed Detox Water

Ingredients :

- Chia seeds
- lemon juice
- water, honey

Preparation :

1. Soak chia seeds in water

2. Add lemon juice and honey

3. Drink to cleanse the gut and boost energy.

Ginger Mint Detox Tea

Ingredients :

- Fresh mint leaves
- Ginger
- Hot water.

Preparation :

1. Steep mint and ginger in hot water

2. Strain and drink to soothe digestion and reduce bloating.

Aloe Vera Cleanse Drink

Ingredients:

- Aloe vera gel
- Lemon juice
- Water

Preparation:

1. Blend aloe vera gel with lemon juice and water

2. Drink to support the digestive system.

Spirulina Detox Smoothie

Ingredients:

- Spirulina powder
- Banana
- Spinach
- Almond milk

Preparation:

1. Blend all ingredients for a smoothie that cleanses while providing a boost of nutrients.

Cucumber Lemon Detox Water

Ingredients:

- Cucumber
- Lemon
- Water

Preparation:

1. Slice cucumber and lemon, add to water and infuse overnight to detoxify and promote hydration.

Broccoli Detox Soup

Ingredients:

- Broccoli
- Onions
- Celery
- Vegetable broth
- Garlic

Preparation :

1. Cook all ingredients until tender

2. Blend into a soup that supports detoxification through cruciferous vegetables.

Kale and Apple Detox Salad

Ingredients :

- Kale
- Green apple
- Walnuts
- Lemon dressing

Preparation :

1. Mix chopped kale and apple

2. Add walnuts

3. Toss with lemon dressing for a detoxifying salad.

Flaxseed Detox Breakfast Bowl

Ingredients :

- Ground flaxseed
- Almond milk
- Berries
- Banana

Preparation :

1. Mix flaxseed with almond milk

2. Top with berries and banana for a fiber-rich breakfast that aids detox.

Pomegranate Detox Tea

Ingredients :

- Pomegranate seeds
- Green tea
- Hot water

Preparation :

1. Brew green tea

2. Add pomegranate seeds

3. Drink to benefit from antioxidants and detox properties.

Seaweed Salad

Ingredients :

- Seaweed
- Cucumber
- Sesame seeds
- Soy sauce
- Rice vinegar

Preparation :

1. Soak seaweed

2. Mix with cucumber and sesame seeds

3. Dress with soy sauce and vinegar for a nutrient-dense detox salad.

Golden Milk

Ingredients :

- Turmeric
- Coconut milk
- Black pepper
- Honey

Preparation :

1. Heat coconut milk

2. Add turmeric and a pinch of black pepper

3. Sweeten with honey and drink to reduce inflammation.

Avocado Detox Smoothie

Ingredients :

- Avocado
- Spinach
- Cucumber
- Lemon juice

Preparation :

1. Blend all ingredients for a creamy

2. Detoxifying smoothie.

Pineapple and Basil Detox Water

Ingredients :

- Pineapple
- Basil leaves
- Water

Preparation :

1. Combine chopped pineapple and basil in water

2. Infuse to create a detoxifying and refreshing drink.

Red Beet Detox Smoothie

Ingredients :

- Cooked beets
- carrot
- ginger
- apple
- lemon juice

Preparation :

1. Blend all ingredients to make a liver-supportive detox smoothie

Lemon and Cayenne Pepper Cleanse

Ingredients :

- Lemon juice
- Cayenne pepper
- Maple syrup
- Water

Preparation :

1. Mix all ingredients and drink to stimulate digestion and cleanse the system.

These recipes provide a variety of options for incorporating detoxifying foods and drinks into your daily routine, helping to cleanse the body and promote optimal health.

25 Healthy Organic Recipes

Explore 25 wholesome recipes that utilize whole, nutrient-dense ingredients to craft delicious and nourishing meals. Dive into these healthy creations for a revitalized eating experience.

Quinoa and Black Bean Salad

Ingredients :

- Quinoa
- Black beans
- Tomatoes
- Avocado
- Lime dressing

Preparation :

1. Cook quinoa

2. Mix with rinsed black beans

3. Chopped tomatoes and avocado

4. Dress with lime juice

5. Olive oil

6. Salt

7. Pepper

Roasted Sweet Potato and Kale Bowl

Ingredients :

- Sweet potatoes
- Kale
- Quinoa
- Pumpkin seeds
- Tahini dressing

Preparation :

1. Roast sweet potatoes

2. Sauté kale

3. Serve over quinoa

4. Top with pumpkin seeds and drizzle with tahini dressing.

Vegetarian Lentil Soup

Ingredients:

- Lentils
- Carrots
- Onions
- Celery
- Tomatoes
- Vegetable broth

Preparation:

1. Cook all ingredients until lentils are tender

2. Season with herbs and spices to taste.

Spiced Chickpea Wraps

Ingredients:

- Chickpeas
- Whole wheat tortillas
- Mixed greens
- Yogurt
- Cumin
- Paprika

Preparation:

1. Toss chickpeas with cumin and paprika

2. Roast until crispy

3. Wrap in tortillas with greens and a dollop of yogurt.

Avocado Toast with Poached Egg

Ingredients :

- Whole grain bread
- Avocado
- Eggs
- Vinegar

Preparation :

1. Toast bread

2. Mash avocado on top

3. Poach eggs in water with a little vinegar

4. Place eggs on avocado toast

Grilled Salmon with Mango Salsa

Ingredients :

- Salmon fillets
- Mango
- Red bell pepper
- Red onion
- Cilantro
- Lime

Preparation :

1. Grill salmon

2. Mix diced mango

3. Bell pepper

4. Onion

5. Cilantro

6. Lime juice for salsa

7. Serve together

Stuffed Bell Peppers

Ingredients:

- Bell peppers
- Brown rice
- Black beans
- Corn
- Tomatoes
- Cheese

Preparation:

1. Halve and seed peppers

2. Stuff with cooked rice

3. Beans

4. Corn

5. Tomatoes

6. Top with cheese

7. Bake until peppers are tender

Butternut Squash Soup

Ingredients:

- Butternut squash
- Onions
- Vegetable broth
- Coconut milk
- Spices

Preparation:

1. Roast squash

2. Sauté onions

3. Blend all ingredients until smooth

4. Simmer to combine flavors.

Kale and Apple Salad with Walnut Dressing

Ingredients :

- Kale
- Apple
- Walnuts
- Cider vinegar
- Olive oil
- Mustard

Preparation :

1. Chop kale and apple

2. Blend walnuts with vinegar

3. Oil

4. Mustard for dressing

5. Toss everything together

Broccoli and Chickpea Stir-Fry

Ingredients :

- Broccoli
- Chickpeas
- Garlic
- Soy sauce
- Sesame oil.

Preparation :

1. Stir-fry broccoli and chickpeas with garlic

2. Finish with soy sauce and a drizzle of sesame oil.

Beet and Goat Cheese Arugula Salad

Ingredients :

- Beets
- Goat cheese
- Arugula
- Balsamic vinegar
- Olive oil.

Preparation :

1. Roast beets

2. slice and serve on arugula with crumbled goat cheese

3. dress with balsamic and olive oil

Oatmeal Banana Pancakes

Ingredients :

- Rolled oats
- Bananas
- Eggs
- Baking powder
- Cinnamon

Preparation :

1. Blend all ingredients to make batter

2. Cook pancakes on a hot griddle until golden.

Mediterranean Quinoa Salad

Ingredients :

- Quinoa
- Cucumber
- Kalamata olives
- Feta cheese
- Lemon dressing

Preparation :

1. Cook quinoa

2. Mix with chopped cucumber

3. Olives

4. Feta

5. Dress with lemon juice and olive oil.

Tomato Basil Pasta

Ingredients :

- Whole wheat pasta
- Fresh tomatoes
- Basil
- Garlic
- Olive oil

Preparation :

1. Cook pasta

2. Sauté garlic and chopped tomatoes in olive oil

3. Toss with pasta and fresh basil.

Curried Cauliflower Rice

Ingredients :

- Cauliflower
- Onions

- Curry powder
- Peas
- Coconut oil

Preparation:

1. Grate cauliflower into 'rice'

2. Sauté with onions and curry powder in coconut oil

3. Peas

4. Cook until tender

Pumpkin Spice Smoothie

Ingredients:

- Pumpkin puree
- Banana
- Almond milk
- Pumpkin spice
- Maple syrup

Preparation:

1. Blend all ingredients until smooth for a seasonal treat

Spinach and Feta Stuffed Chicken

Ingredients:

- Chicken breasts
- Spinach
- Feta cheese
- Garlic

Preparation:

1. Stuff chicken with sautéed spinach and feta

2. bake until chicken is cooked through

Sweet Potato and Black Bean Tacos

Ingredients :

- Sweet potatoes
- Black beans
- Corn tortillas
- Avocado
- Lime crema

Preparation :

1. Roast sweet potatoes

2. Serve in tortillas with black beans and sliced avocado

3. Top with lime crema

Zucchini Noodles with Pesto

Ingredients :

- Zucchini
- Basil
- Garlic
- Pine nuts
- Parmesan cheese
- Olive oil

Preparation :

1. Spiralize zucchini

2. Bend basil

3. Garlic

4. Nuts

5. Cheese

6. Oil for pesto

7. Toss zoodles with pesto

Cauliflower Steak with Herb Sauce

Ingredients:

- Cauliflower
- Parsley
- Cilantro
- Garlic
- Lemon
- Olive oil.

Preparation:

1. Slice cauliflower into steaks

2. Roast until tender

3. Blend herbs with garlic

4. Lemon

5. Oil for sauce

Mushroom Risotto

Ingredients:

- Arborio rice
- Mushrooms
- Onions
- Vegetable broth
- Parmesan cheese

Preparation:

1. Sauté mushrooms and onions

2. Add rice

3. Gradually add broth

4. Stirring until creamy

5. Finish with cheese

Chickpea and Vegetable Curry

Ingredients :

- Chickpeas
- Coconut milk
- Curry paste
- Mixed vegetables

Preparation :

1. Sauté vegetables

2. Add curry paste

3. Chickpeas

4. Coconut milk

5. Simmer until vegetables are tender.

Apple Cinnamon Overnight Oats

Ingredients :

- Rolled oats
- Almond milk
- Apple
- Cinnamon
- Honey

Preparation :

1. Mix oats with milk

2. Chopped apple

3. Cinnamon

4. Honey

5. Let sit overnight in the fridge.

Baked Cod with Lemon and Dill

Ingredients :

- Cod fillets
- Lemon
- Dill
- Olive oil

Preparation :

1. Place cod in a baking dish

2. Season with lemon slices

3. Dill

4. Olive oil

5. Bake until fish flakes easily

Asian Tofu Stir-Fry

Ingredients :

- Tofu
- Bell peppers
- Broccoli
- Soy sauce
- Ginger
- Garlic

Preparation :

1. Sauté tofu until golden

2. Add vegetables and stir-fry with ginger and garlic

3. Finish with soy sauce

These healthy organic recipes emphasize the use of fresh, unprocessed ingredients to create meals that are both nourishing and flavorful, suitable for anyone looking to maintain a healthy diet.

25 Herbal Teas and Infusions

Discover 25 herbal teas and infusions, each selected for their remarkable health benefits and therapeutic properties. Enjoy these soothing brews for enhanced well-being.

Chamomile Tea

Benefits :

- Calms the nervous system
- Aids sleep
- Reduces inflammation

Preparation :

- Steep dried chamomile flowers in hot water for 5-10 minutes

Peppermint Tea

Benefits :

- Soothes digestion
- Relieves headaches
- Enhances focus

Preparation :

- Infuse fresh or dried peppermint leaves in boiling water for 5-7 minutes

Ginger Tea

Benefits :

- Stimulates digestion
- Relieves nausea
- Fights inflammation

Preparation :

- Simmer slices of fresh ginger root in water for 10-15 minutes

Hibiscus Tea

Benefits:

- Lowers blood pressure
- Antioxidant-rich
- Supports liver health

Preparation:

- Steep dried hibiscus flowers in boiling water for 5 minutes

Green Tea

Benefits:

- Rich in antioxidants
- enhances brain function
- promotes fat loss

Preparation:

- Steep green tea leaves in hot water (not boiling) for 2-3 minutes

Rooibos Tea

Benefits:

- Caffeine-free
- High in antioxidants
- Supports heart health

Preparation:

- Steep rooibos leaves in boiling water for 5-7 minutes

Lemon Balm Tea

Benefits :

- Reduces anxiety
- Supports sleep
- Eases indigestion

Preparation :

- Infuse dried lemon balm leaves in boiling water for 5-10 minutes

Nettle Tea

Benefits :

- Rich in nutrients
- Supports joint health
- Aids detoxification

Preparation :

- Steep dried nettle leaves in hot water for 10-15 minutes

Dandelion Root Tea

Benefits :

- Detoxifies the liver
- Promotes digestion
- Reduces water retention

Preparation :

- Simmer dried dandelion root in water for 5-10 minutes

Lavender Tea

Benefits :

- Reduces stress
- aids sleep
- supports skin health

Preparation :

- Infuse dried lavender flowers in boiling water for 5-7 minutes

Fennel Seed Tea

Benefits :

- Supports digestion
- Relieves bloating
- Provides antioxidants

Preparation :

- Crush fennel seeds slightly
- Steep in boiling water for 5-10 minutes

Licorice Root Tea

Benefits :

- Soothes the stomach
- supports adrenal function
- relieves sore throat

Preparation :

- Simmer slices of licorice root in water for 10-15 minutes.

Echinacea Tea

Benefits :

- Boosts the immune system and fights colds and flu

Preparation :

- Steep echinacea root or flowers in hot water for 10-15 minutes

Yerba Mate

Benefits :

- Increases energy
- Enhances mental focus
- Contains antioxidants

Preparation :

- Steep yerba mate leaves in hot water for 5-7 minutes

Sage Tea

Benefits :

- Supports brain health
- Alleviates sore throats
- Regulates digestion

Preparation :

- Steep dried sage leaves in boiling water for about 5-7 minutes.

Tulsi Tea (Holy Basil)

Benefits :

- Reduces stress
- Supports the immune system
- Balances energy levels

Preparation :

- Infuse tulsi leaves in hot water for about 5-8 minutes

Spearmint Tea

Benefits :

- Aids digestion
- Relieves nausea
- Has hormone-balancing properties

Preparation :

- Steep dried spearmint leaves in boiling water for 5 minutes

Rose Hip Tea

Benefits :

- High in Vitamin C
- Supports immune health
- Aids skin and tissue health

Preparation :

- Steep crushed rose hips in hot water for about 10-15 minutes

Passionflower Tea

Benefits :

- Promotes relaxation
- Supports sleep
- Reduces anxiety

Preparation :

- Infuse dried passionflower in boiling water for 10 minutes

Valerian Root Tea

Benefits :

- Aids sleep
- reduces anxiety
- helps in managing stress

Preparation :

- Simmer valerian root in water for 10 minutes before drinking at bedtime

Cinnamon Tea

Benefits :

- Balances blood sugar
- Improves digestion
- Has anti - inflammatory properties

Preparation :

- Boil cinnamon sticks in water for 15-20 minutes.

Cardamom Tea

Benefits :

- Aids digestion
- Stimulates metabolism
- Has detoxifying properties

Preparation :

- Crush cardamom pods
- Steep in boiling water for 10 minutes

Mullein Tea

Benefits :

- Supports respiratory health
- Relieves coughs
- Reduces inflammation

Preparation :

- Steep dried mullein leaves and flowers in boiling water for about 10 minutes.

Burdock Root Tea

Benefits :

- Detoxifies the blood
- Supports liver health
- Aids skin health

Preparation :

- Simmer dried burdock root in water for about 10 minutes.

Marshmallow Root Tea

Benefits :

- Soothes the digestive tract
- Relieves irritation of the mucous membranes
- Aids in healing ulcers

Preparation :

- Steep dried marshmallow root in cold water for several hours

These herbal teas and infusions offer a range of therapeutic benefits, making them excellent choices for those seeking natural ways to enhance health and well-being.

25 Specialty Remedies and Treatments

Explore 25 specialty remedies and treatments, each designed with natural and alternative approaches to specifically address health concerns and boost overall wellness.

Cold and Flu Bomb

Ingredients :

- Garlic
- Ginger
- Lemon
- Honey
- Cayenne pepper

Preparation :

1. Blend all ingredients into a potent syrup to take at the first sign of cold symptoms.

Herbal Pain Relief Salve

Ingredients :

- Cayenne pepper
- Ginger
- Beeswax
- Coconut oil.

Preparation :

1. Infuse oils with cayenne and ginger

2. Mix with melted beeswax to form a salve

3. Apply topically for pain relief

Natural Sleep Aid Tincture

Ingredients :

- Valerian root
- Hops
- Alcohol

Preparation :

1. Macerate valerian and hops in alcohol for several weeks to create a potent tincture for insomnia.

Digestive Bitters

Ingredients:

- Dandelion root
- Gentian root
- Orange peel
- Alcohol

Preparation:

1. Combine ingredients in alcohol

2. Let steep

3. Use before meals to aid digestion.

Anti-Anxiety Herbal Blend

Ingredients:

- Lavender
- Chamomile
- Lemon balm

Preparation:

4. Mix herbs in equal parts to make a tea or tincture to help soothe anxiety.

Throat Soothing Syrup

Ingredients:

- Marshmallow root
- Licorice root
- Honey
- Water

Preparation:

1. Simmer roots in water

2. Strain

3. Add honey

4. Take as needed for sore throat relief.

Herbal Antifungal Powder

Ingredients :

- Arrowroot powder
- Tea tree oil
- Neem powder

Preparation :

1. Mix ingredients and apply to affected areas to combat fungal infections

Detoxifying Bath Soak

Ingredients :

- Epsom salts
- Baking soda
- Lavender oil
- Ground ginger

Preparation :

1. Mix all ingredients and add to a warm bath to help detoxify the body and relax muscles.

Immunity Boosting Tonic

Ingredients :

- Echinacea
- Elderberry
- Astragalus
- Water
- Honey

Preparation :

1. Simmer herbs in water

2. Strain

3. Add honey

4. Drink regularly to boost the immune system.

Migraine Relief Oil Blend

Ingredients :

- Peppermint oil
- Lavender o
- Coconut oil

Preparation :

1. Mix essential oils with coconut oil and apply to temples and neck during migraine attacks.

Natural Decongestant Steam

Ingredients :

- Eucalyptus oil
- Peppermint oil
- Hot water

Preparation :

1. Add essential oils to boiling water and inhale steam to clear nasal passages.

Homemade Electrolyte Drink

Ingredients :

- Lemon juice
- Water
- Honey
- Sea salt

Preparation :

1. Mix all ingredients to replenish fluids and electrolytes after dehydration

Calming Magnesium Drink

Ingredients :

- Magnesium citrate powder
- Water
- Lemon juice

Preparation :

1. Dissolve magnesium powder in water

2. Add lemon for taste

3. Drink at night to promote relaxation.

Wound Healing Poultice

Ingredients :

- Comfrey leaves
- Water

Preparation :

1. Blend comfrey leaves with a little water to make a paste

2. Apply directly to wounds to speed healing.

Anti-Inflammatory Golden Paste

Ingredients :

- Turmeric
- Black pepper
- Coconut oil

Preparation :

1. Cook turmeric with water to form a paste

2. Add black pepper and coconut oil

3. Consume daily

Soothing Skin Balm

Ingredients:

- Calendula
- Shea butter
- Beeswax
- Almond oil

Preparation:

1. Infuse almond oil with calendula

2. Mix with melted shea butter and beeswax

3. Cool to form a balm for skin irritations

Liver Detox Tea

Ingredients:

- Milk thistle
- Burdock root
- Dandelion root.

Preparation:

1. Steep herbs in hot water to create a tea that supports liver detoxification.

Stress Relief Aroma Inhaler

Ingredients:

- Bergamot oil
- Frankincense oil
- Sandalwood oil

Preparation:

1. Add essential oils to a personal aroma inhaler to use during stressful times.

Menstrual Cramp Relief Oil

Ingredients :

- Clary sage oil
- Lavender oil
- Coconut oil.

Preparation :

1. Mix essential oils with coconut oil and apply to the abdomen to relieve menstrual cramps.

Joint Pain Liniment

Ingredients :

- Arnica
- Cayenne
- Apple cider
- Vinegar
- Alcohol

Preparation :

1. Macerate arnica and cayenne in a mixture of vinegar and alcohol

2. Apply externally to painful joints.

Memory Boosting Syrup

Ingredients :

- Ginkgo biloba
- Rosemary
- Water
- Honey

Preparation:

1. Simmer ginkgo and rosemary in water

2. Strain

3. Add honey

4. Take daily to enhance memory and cognitive function.

Natural Laxative Formula

Ingredients:

- Senna leaves
- Fennel seeds
- Ginger

Preparation:

1. Combine herbs in equal parts

2. Steep in boiling water

3. Drink to relieve constipation.

Breath Freshening Herbal Chew

Ingredients:

- Parsley
- Mint
- Cloves

Preparation:

1. Chop herbs

2. Mix with cloves

3. Chew after meals to freshen breath

Anti-Aging Skin Serum

Ingredients:

- Rosehip seed oil
- Frankincense oil
- Vitamin E.

Preparation:

1. Mix oils with vitamin E

2. Apply to the face at night for its regenerative properties.

These specialty remedies and treatments offer targeted, natural solutions for a variety of health concerns, utilizing the healing powers of herbs, essential oils, and other natural ingredients.

CONCLUSION

After exploring Barbara's teachings and insights, it is important to pause and reflect on what we have learned.

We should consider which steps we still need to take in our lives and how they will lead to outcomes. This book serves as a guide helping us understand how to improve our well being, increase our lifespan, heal ourselves and experience vitality.

Let's pause for a moment.

Appreciate the journey this book represents. We have delved into the "Foundation of Health". We discussed nutrition, sleep patterns, sunlight exposure, and physical activity. Barbara has provided us with detailed guidelines in these areas. Additionally we've explored natural remedies and concluded with detailed explanations of various recipes. My hope is that this book can help you grasp Barbara's insights and make an impact on your life.

All the best,
Lane Snyder

Made in the USA
Las Vegas, NV
04 May 2024

89542767R00109